The Effective Management of Lung Cancer

Second edition

The Effective Management of Lung Cancer

Second edition

Edited by

Martin Muers MA DPhil FRCP
Consultant Physician & Chairman, British Thoracic Society Lung Cancer Working Party,
The General Infirmary at Leeds, Leeds, UK

Nicholas Thatcher PhD FRCP
Professor of Oncology, The Christie Hospital, Manchester, UK

Francis Wells MB BS MA MS FRCS
Consultant Cardiothoracic Surgeon, Papworth Hospital, Cambridge, UK

Andrew Miles MSc MPhil PhD
Professor of Public Health Sciences, Barts and The London,
Queen Mary's School of Medicine and Dentistry, University of London, UK

Barts and The London
Queen Mary's School of
Medicine and Dentistry

Association of
Cancer
Physicians

The Royal College
of
Radiologists

Society of
Cardiothoracic
Surgeons

British
Thoracic
Society

AESCULAPIUS MEDICAL PRESS
LONDON SAN FRANCISCO SYDNEY

Published by

Aesculapius Medical Press (London, San Francisco, Sydney)
P. O. Box LB48
London EC1A 1LB, UK

© Aesculapius Medical Press 2003

First published 2003

British Library Cataloguing in Publication Data
A catalogue record for this book is available from the British Library

ISBN 1 903044 28 6

While the advice and information in this book are believed to be true and accurate at the
time of going to press, neither the authors nor the editors nor the sponsoring institutions
can accept any legal responsibility or liability for any errors or omissions that may be made.
In particular (but without limiting the generality of the preceding disclaimer) every effort
has been made to check drug usages; however, it is possible that errors have been missed.
Furthermore, dosage schedules are constantly being revised and new side effects recognised.
For these reasons, the reader is strongly urged to consult the drug companies' printed
instructions before administering any of the drugs discussed in this book.

Further copies of this book are available from:

Claudio Melchiorri
Research Dissemination Fellow
Key Advances Ltd
P. O. Box LB48
London EC1A 1LB, UK

Fax: 020 – 8525 – 8661
e-mail: claudio@keyadvances4.demon.co.uk

Typeset, printed and bound in Britain
Peter Powell Origination & Print Limited

Contents

Contributors

Jesme Baird MB ChB MBA, Director of Patient Care, Roy Castle Lung Cancer Foundation, Glasgow

DR Baldwin MD FRCP, Consultant Respiratory Physician, Nottingham City Hospital, Nottingham.

Michael Cullen BSc MD FRCR FRCP, Consultant Oncologist, Queen Elizabeth Hospital, Birmingham

RJ Fergusson MD FRCP, Consultant Respiratory Physician, Western General Hospital, Edinburgh

David Gibbs MB ChB FRACP, Clinical Research Fellow, Royal Marsden Hospital, London and Surrey

Peter Goldstraw FRCS, Consultant Thoracic Surgeon, Royal Brompton Hospital, London

Anna Gregor FRCR FRCP, Consultant Clinical Oncologist and Lead Cancer Clinician for Scotland, Western General Hospital, Edinburgh

Janet ES Husband FRCR FRCP FMedSci, Professor of Diagnostic Radiology, Royal Marsden Hospital, London and Surrey

G Jayson BA BM BCh PhD MRCP, Senior Lecturer in Medical Oncology & Honorary Consultant Medical Oncologist, Christie Hospital, Manchester

Sarah Khan MB ChB MD MRCP, Specialist Registrar in Medical Oncology, City Hospital, Nottingham

Mary O'Brien MD FRCP, Consultant Medical Oncologist, Royal Marsden Hospital, London and Surrey

Andreas Polychronis MB MRCP, Specialist Registrar/Clinical Research Fellow in Medical Oncology, Imperial College at the Hammersmith Hospital, London

Malcolm Ranson MB ChB PhD MRCP, Senior Lecturer in Medical Oncology & Honorary Consultant Medical Oncologist, Christie Hospital, Manchester

Robin M Rudd MD FRCP, Consultant Medical Oncologist, St. Bartholomew's Hospital, London

Michele I Saunders MD FRCR FRCP, Professor of Clinical Oncology, University College London and Consultant Clinical Oncologist, Mount Vernon Hospital, Middlesex

Jeremy PC Steele MD MRCP, Consultant Medical Oncologist, St. Bartholomew's Hospital, London

Nicholas Thatcher PhD FRCP, Professor of Oncology, Christie Hospital, Manchester and Wythenshawe Hospital, Manchester

Nicholas Wald FFPHM FRCP FMedSci, Professor, Wolfson Institute of Preventive Medicine, Charterhouse Square, London

Francis Wells MB BS MA MS FRCS, Consultant Cardiothoracic Surgeon, Papworth Hospital, Cambridge

Penella J Woll PhD FRCP, Professor of Medical Oncology, University of Sheffield

Preface

The prognosis for patients with lung cancer remains poor with the overall 5-year survival rates varying from 12–15% in the USA, for example, to 5% in Scotland. Survival rates are strongly related to the stage of the disease at the time of diagnosis and while surgery remains the best treatment option for established disease, less than 20% of tumours are suitable for potentially curative resection and only about 30% of these survive for five years. Advances in molecular biology have opened up enormous possibilities to identify individuals who are at risk of developing lung cancer, an observation which may be considered at two levels: the ability to identify individuals who are at risk because of their genetic background and the ability to identify individuals who are at risk because of their exposure to carcinogens during their lifetime. Chemoprevention has, within these contexts, therefore to be recognised as a future clinical option and the time has probably come to develop chemopreventive strategies in tandem with developments in molecular genetic early detection techniques. Such a thesis appears in many ways unarguable in a country such as the UK where lung cancer accounts for approximately 40,000 deaths per annum.

While advances in molecular genetics continue to be made with encouraging frequency, their clinical applications have yet to be fully worked out and this is likely to remain the case for some years to come. However, the application of more recently piloted screening techniques may be considered of more immediate relevance to early diagnosis and effective treatment. The effect of lung cancer screening remains most appropriately demonstrated by randomised controlled trials with disease specific mortality as the primary endpoint and while the results of such trials in the 1970s (based on chest radiography and sputum cytology) demonstrated no obvious survival benefits, more recent studies from non-randomised designs in Japan and the United States of America using spiral CT as the screening technology have shown encouraging results, in the majority of patients the disease being early stage.

It is noteworthy in this context that surgery in patients whose disease has been detected at stage I results in 5-year survival rates ranging between 55–70% and so the next logical step, as Husband and Wald outline, is for a randomised trial to be conducted of spiral CT screening versus no screening in smokers, aged 60 years or over, with lung cancer mortality employed as the primary end point. The authors proceed to describe such a study design and argue how, if a positive result were to be achieved in such a trial, the health benefits from targeted application of the technology would be as great or indeed even greater than those shown for breast cancer screening.

The second part of the volume, through chapters 2 and 3, examines the evidence base for surgical intervention in established disease. Any manoeuvre which is designed to reduce the *perceived* extent of disease as assessed by the clinical TNM stage prior to the institution of definitive treatment, may be described as 'downstaging' and it is to this initial therapy that Goldstraw turns. As he points out, our perception of the extent of disease prior to treatment, cTNM, is dependent first upon the subjective interpretation of data (largely deriving from imaging techniques) and second on the results from the published literature on induction therapy being largely derived from heterogenous patient populations. As a consequence there are conflicting opinions on the value of induction treatment prior to surgery. Certainly, strong evidence is lacking which suggests that induction therapy can render irresectable disease resectable or that medically inoperable cases can be rendered operable by reducing the extent of disease.

If induction therapy is to improve prognosis in inoperable cases then it must include chemotherapy in order to eradicate micrometastatic disease and there are considerable resource implications associated with this approach. Whether such treatment can improve prognosis is not yet definitively known and induction therapy may simply mislead us by altering only the state of intrathoracic prognostic indicators (e.g. lymph nodes) and not by effecting any real benefits to the patient. Questions such as these will begin to be answered, however, by prospective randomised controlled trials with some of these actively recruiting and others being considered. In this situation it may well be, as Goldstraw feels, appropriate to concentrate more specifically on the extended provision of thoracic surgery in order to ensure that cases that are operable by conventional criteria receive specialist intervention as early as possible.

Wells concentrates on the provision of appropriate surgery, specifically on the place of extended resection and reconstructive surgery. Tumours involving direct invasion of the chest wall and/or diaphragm have long been recognised as being operable and the aim of surgery has therefore been complete resection. It has always been recognised that mediastinal node involvement precludes cure but direct mediastinal node involvement in selected cases such as pericardial invasion with left atrial encroachment continue to be considered resectable (in contrast to direct mediastinal invasion of the superior vena cava or aorta) although with varying long term but probably acceptable midterm, survival. It is becoming more widely accepted that locally advanced disease within the chest in the absence of mediastinal node spread can be treated surgically. Undoubtedly, in the modern era of cardiothoracic surgery, such resections are increasingly possible with increasingly satisfactory postoperative outcomes. However, the real impact of this type of surgery in locally advanced tumours, as the author points out, awaits availability of good quality, peer reviewed prospectively gathered evidence.

Having considered the possible benefits of novel screening methods in Part 1, and Part 2 having reviewed the benefits of surgical intervention, Part 3 of the text, through chapters 4, 5 and 6, is dedicated to a review of the scientific evidence underpinning medical intervention in established disease. Saunders, in the initial chapter of this section, provides a thorough review of the place of CHART, CHARTWEL and combined modalities. The CHART schedule of radiotherapy was introduced to overcome cellular re-population in tumours during the prolonged course of conventional radiotherapy. It proved possible to reduce the duration of radiotherapy from 42 days to 12 days and in a randomised controlled trial conducted between 1990 and 1995 comparing CHART to conventional radiotherapy, CHART provided a significant benefit in terms of survival, local recurrence and disease-free interval with the benefit being estimated at twice that which had been reported as given by the addition of chemotherapy. CHART was therefore recommended by the NHS Executive as the treatment of choice for early inoperable non-small cell lung cancer. However, the implementation of the protocol (which requires radiotherapy three times a day inclusive of weekends) has, as Saunders discusses, proved difficult and only six UK centres at the time of writing are now offering this regimen, despite the clear evidence of its superior effectiveness.

Not surprisingly, perhaps, the major obstacles are, as the author points out, a lack of linear accelerators and skilled radiographers and the difficulties associated with weekend working in the UK National Health Service. In order to address these deficiencies the CHARTWEL regimen (CHART weekend-less) has been formulated and at Mount Vernon Hospital, Middlesex, UK, has been introduced in phase I/II dose escalation studies and by extending into the third week it has proved possible to elevate the total radiation dose. Both in Germany and the UK, CHARTWEL to 60Gy over seventeen days treating three times per day has shown promise in phase II studies and radiobiological modelling suggests that the increase in dose will increase the local tumour control achieved with CHART by between 4 and 20% without a significant increase in early or late morbidity. The addition of chemotherapy can also give benefit and so the way forward, Saunders argues, is to combine CHART or CHARTWEL with neoadjuvant and/or concomitant chemotherapy in a further effort to improve results. These studies, exploring new regimens of neoadjuvant and concurrent chemotherapy, are currently being conducted.

Most patients with lung cancer will die with disseminated disease and so it is logical to use systemic therapy as early as possible in the course of the disease in order to treat micrometastases. In other tumour types, adjuvant and neoadjuvant chemotherapy have substantially improved the cure rates obtained by surgery or radiotherapy alone but in non-small cell lung cancer the role of chemotherapy in early stage disease has been questioned over the course of the last thirty years of research. In chapter 5, Khan and Woll examine the data that has accumulated to date for the effectiveness of chemotherapy in early disease. In a meta-analysis of data from 9387 patients involved in 52 randomised controlled trials the effect of chemotherapy when combined with local treatment (surgery or radiotherapy) demonstrated that the addition of alkylating agents to either surgery or radiotherapy was detrimental although for cisplatin-containing regimens there was a small but significant survival advantage from chemotherapy. The subsequent studies reviewed by the authors are shown to confirm these earlier results with a potential 10%

improvement in 5-year survival rates for combined modality treatments. The role of newer agents such as docetaxel, paclitaxel, gemcitabine, vinorelbine and topoisomerase inhibitors remains under careful evaluation.

In chapter 6, the concluding chapter of this section, Gibbs, O'Brien and Polychronis are similarly concerned to evaluate the effects of chemotherapy in lung cancer but in the context of first and second line intervention in advanced disease. There is, as the authors point out, Level 1a evidence for a small benefit from palliative chemotherapy in non-small cell lung cancer. Each of the four newer agents, docetaxel, paclitaxel, gemcitabine and vinorelbine has been tested with superior results against no chemotherapy in the first line setting such that the use of any one of these agents in combination with a platinum compound is now appropriate for patients of performance status 0,1 giving survival figures of around 30% at one year. Of the newer compounds, docetaxel is currently the only agent which has been compared to no chemotherapy in the second line setting with a statistically significant survival advantage being documented. This has led to suggestions that docetaxel should be employed in patients with a good performance status who have been platinum sensitive although its effectiveness in patients with PS 2 and primary platinum resistance remains the subject of further investigation.

There is little doubt that further clinical trials are necessary to develop our understanding of the potential of the existing newer chemotherapies in early and advanced disease and to test the usefulness of the newer, so called biological agents and Part 4 of the volume, the penultimate section, is dedicated to a detailed discussion of current clinical trials and novel therapies. In the opening chapter, chapter 7, Steele and Rudd define the important questions that remain largely unanswered in relation to the management of lung cancer and proceed to catalogue the existing trials which have been designed to provide additional information for the treatment of the disease. What, for example, is the value of pre-operative chemotherapy in NSCLC? Does postoperative chemotherapy or radiotherapy increase the chance of cure? What is the best treatment for locally advanced but unresectable NSCLC? What is the best treatment for advanced NSCLC?

New cytostatic agents that act on novel cellular targets are emerging and are entering clinical trials. Examples include epidermal growth factor receptor inhibitors, anti-Ras antisense oligonucleotides, farnesyl transferase inhibitors and vascular endothelial growth factor receptor antibodies with an older drug thalidomide having been 're-discovered' and appearing to have a variety of actions of importance for NSCLC, including antiangiogenesis.

It is to biological approaches to the management of disease that Ranson, Jayson and Thatcher turn in chapter 8. Within the context of this work, the point is made that although non-specific cytotoxic drugs have brought significant advances in the treatment of many tumours, it seems increasingly clear that the point of diminishing return has been reached for non-selective cytotoxic drugs in the treatment of many common epithelial tumours, including lung cancer. The recent development of highly selective, target-based cancer therapeutics is likely to transform oncology in the next two decades. Indeed, dose-toxicity relationships may be less steep and therapeutic windows wider than for cytotoxics, rendering traditional endpoints such as maximum tolerable dose (MTD) in phase I trials less relevant with the altered emphasis focusing on more meaningful indices such as the identification of biologically active dose ranges and an attempt to define an optimal biological dose. For phase II trials of cytotoxic anticancer drugs, one important endpoint has been the proportion of patients showing *tumour regression*, the so called response rate (RR). This endpoint is similarly likely to become less relevant in the evaluation of novel target-specific agents. Instead, endpoints that reflect *tumour control* such as time to tumour progression, survival, quality of life and improvement in disease-related symptoms are required. For phase III trials techniques that allow early readout of biological effect using direct or surrogate measurements, for example, biopsy assessment of drug target inhibition, positron emission tomography and dynamic MR, may become increasingly important. The authors are clear that while it is certainly true that the rational development of these novel agents will require substantial investment in translational research, the potential for tumour management and disease prevention within individuals identified at high risk, is exciting indeed.

The final section of the volume, Part 5, is dedicated to a discussion of core issues in the provision of clinical services. There is, as Cullen points out in chapter 9, a strong feeling and some evidence that lung cancer remains inadequately investigated and treated in the UK. For this author, the evidence consists of low rates of histological verification of disease, substantial regional variations in surgical resection, utilisation of chemotherapy and survival relative to other developed countries. The reasons which underpin these observations, the author asserts, include ignorance about the disease and what can be achieved with optimal treatment, prejudice among some professional groups against active intervention, the perceived and actual cost of optimal treatment, a shortage of sufficient radiotherapy equipment, low numbers of dedicated lung cancer surgeons, oncologists, specialist nurses and radiographers, a system which until recently was not conducive to multidisciplinary decision making and a notoriously undemanding and unassertive patient population. Following Cullen's discussion of these matters and the broad implications of the judgements made by the National Institute for Clinical Excellence (NICE) for the scale of demand for chemotherapy in NSCLC, Fergusson and Gregor outline, in chapter 10, the approaches taken by Government to address many of the difficulties and deficiencies identified through the UK as a whole but with a particular emphasis, in illustration of some important principles and methods, of current progress in Scotland.

In the commentary above we highlighted Cullen's opinion about the undemanding and unassertive nature of the lung cancer patient population. Recently, however, there are encouraging signs that matters are changing. In chapter 11, the penultimate chapter of the book, Baird notes that other disease groups, such as breast cancer patient groups and HIV patient groups, have been highly successful in raising awareness of their disease. This has led to an increase in funding for disease investigation and management and in this way assisting real improvements in the quality and delivery of breast cancer and HIV clinical services. She points out that to date there has been little mobilisation of lung cancer groups for this purpose and reflects on the barriers to such an engagement and what might be done to increase the active participation of patients and their carers in bringing about change. Individual case studies and specific examples may certainly be quoted in support of their potential but a lack of wider knowledge on the most effective strategies to achieve beneficial change is hampering progress. Interestingly, however, the author describes a range of structured initiatives driven by voluntary sector lung cancer patient organisations which are aimed at increasing the media profile and thus public awareness of lung cancer and at increasing the participation of patients' representatives in the work of local services and national organisations. The results of these initiatives will be awaited with much interest.

The systematic audit of the quality of clinical services is a core principle of clinical governance and the final chapter of the volume is dedicated to a detailed discussion of this important activity. As Baldwin points out, accurate measurement of key clinical indicators of service function is essential for successful clinical audit and in recent years there have been a number of developments put in place with the intention of achieving this aim. Nevertheless, a continuing difficulty, as the author sees it, is incompleteness of data collection and a lack of data verification. It is clear that these two functions need to be incorporated into routine practice in order to monitor and develop service delivery and clinical outcomes. The extent to which the National Cancer Minimum Data Set and the information technology being put in place within the UK Cancer Networks will assist this process remains of course to be seen and is likely to be the subject of study in the third and subsequent editions of this volume.

As in the first edition, we have aimed to provide a current, fully referenced text which is as succinct as possible but as comprehensive as necessary within both the context of the overwhelming quantity of clinical information currently available and with due attention to the modern policy requirements of the NHS. Consultants in Respiratory Medicine, Thoracic Surgery, Clinical and Medical Oncology and their trainees will find the volume of direct importance to their clinical practice and we advance it specifically as an excellent tool for this purpose. We anticipate that the book will also prove of use to clinical nurse specialists and oncology pharmacists as a reference text and to managers, planners and commissioners of lung cancer services when in dialogue with their practising colleagues.

In conclusion, we thank AstraZeneca Ltd and Aventis Pharma Ltd for a grant of unconditional educational sponsorship which helped organise a national symposium held with the endorsement of the British Thoracic Society, the Society of Cardiothoracic Surgeons, The Royal College of Radiologists and the Association of Cancer Physicians at The Royal College of Physicians of London at which synopses of the constituent chapters of the current volume were presented. We also thank the Roy Castle Lung Cancer Foundation for its interest in and ongoing support of this annually updated project.

Martin Muers MA DPhil FRCP
Nicholas Thatcher PhD FRCP
Francis Wells MB BS MS FRCS
Andrew Miles MSc MPhil PhD

Acknowledgements

The following colleagues contributed as members of the expert planning committee for the Year 2001/2002 [2nd Update] UK Key Advances Lung Cancer Project: Dr. Fergus Macbeth, Professor Andrew Miles, Dr. Martin Muers, Dr. Marianne Nicholson, Professor Nicholas Thatcher, Mr. Francis Wells.

The contribution of Dr Andreas Polychronis, Clinical Research Fellow/Specialist Registrar in Medical Oncology, Imperial College School of Medicine at the Hammersmith Hospital, London, as secretary to the committee and assistant editor in the preparation of the current volume, is also acknowledged.

PART 1

Screening

Chapter 1

CT-based screening for lung cancer: philosophy, study designs and current trials

Janet E Husband and Nicholas Wald

The concept of screening for lung cancer has stimulated intense debate over several decades, initially as a result of a number of trials using chest radiography and sputum cytology, and then more recently following early reports that low-dose spiral computed tomography (CT) can identify small peripheral lung cancers in asymptomatic individuals (Kaneko et al. 1996; Sone et al. 1998; Henschke et al. 1999; Diederich et al. 2000). These reports of screening with spiral CT have been met with enthusiasm. Several countries throughout the Western World have begun trials of lung cancer screening and others, including the UK, are currently developing detailed proposals.

In the UK there are approximately 35 000 new cases of lung cancer diagnosed annually and the most recent UK statistics in 1999 revealed that lung cancer accounted for 34 240 deaths, which represents 22% of all cancer deaths in the UK (CRC Cancerstats 1999). Mortality from lung cancer has been declining over recent years, yet, in men, it remains the most common cause of cancer mortality and, in women, the number of deaths from lung cancer are second only to those from breast cancer (Lopez 1995). The vast majority of cases are the result of cigarette smoking and most patients present with advanced disease for which the prognosis is poor; 5-year survival rates are no better than 7–14% (Doll et al. 1994; Berrino et al. 1995). However, patients with non-small cell lung cancer, which accounts for about 80% of all lung cancers, might benefit from screening and early detection because surgery for stage I disease results in 5-year survival rates ranging from 55% to 70% (Mountain 1977; Martini et al. 1995; Nesbitt et al. 1995; Shah et al. 1996). Although the results of such surgical series have provided the rationale for lung cancer screening trials, no trial has yet demonstrated that lung cancer screening reduces lung cancer mortality.

Previous lung cancer screening trials

Increasing rates of lung cancer in the 1960s and 1970s led the National Cancer Institute (NCI) to sponsor three large prospective randomised controlled trials (RCTs) of lung cancer screening with chest radiography with or without sputum cytology (Flehinger et al. 1984; Fontana et al. 1986; Tockman 1986). In Czechoslovakia, a fourth large RCT was also conducted (Kubik et al. 1990, 2000).

Although other smaller non-randomised controlled studies of lung cancer screening were undertaken in the 1970s (Nash et al. 1968; Brett 1968; Wilde 1989), most attention has been focused on the results of the four major studies that all compared chest radiography, with or without sputum cytology, with a control group. All of these studies failed to show a statistically significant reduction in lung cancer mortality as a result of screening.

The Mayo Lung Project is, perhaps, the most important of the four studies in that it is the only study that attempted to define a control group with no screening whatsoever. In this trial 9211 men aged over the 45 who were smokers were included; the screened group of 4618 individuals underwent 4-monthly chest radiographs and sputum cytology. More lung cancers were detected in the screened group (206) compared with the control group (160), more cancer patients in the screened group underwent surgery than in the control group and the survival rate of the screened patients was higher. However, lung cancer mortality was not significantly different between the two groups. In the Czech study, more cancers were also found in the screened group compared with the control group (108 vs 82). As with the Mayo Lung Project, the Czech results showed increased survival in the screened group, but no reduction in lung cancer mortality. The results of these four studies did not show a statistically significant effect on lung cancer mortality, but a useful benefit could not be excluded.

The Prostate, Lung, Colon and Ovarian (PLCO) study is an RCT that is currently under way and is funded by the NCI. This trial aims to determine the role of annual chest radiography in screening for lung cancer. The study has been designed with a power of 89% to detect a difference in lung cancer mortality of 10% (Gohagan et al. 1995). The results of this study are expected soon.

Spiral CT for lung cancer screening

The introduction of low-dose spiral CT has reopened the possibility that lung cancer screening may be worthwhile. There are two bodies of opinion. On the one hand, there are those who believe that non-randomised observational studies are sufficient to determine whether lung cancer screening should be introduced. The proponents of this approach argue that lung cancer is an aggressive tumour and is therefore not subject to overdiagnosis and that, in view of these inherent characteristics of the disease, survival can be used as a proxy for mortality. It is argued that non-randomised studies are cheaper and that conclusions from such studies can be drawn more rapidly than from randomised trials. However, non-randomised trials are subject to bias, notably lead-time and length bias, and they do not directly address the question, 'does screening with low-dose spiral CT reduce lung cancer mortality?' Furthermore, there is growing evidence that screen-detected lung cancers may represent a wide range of tumour histologies, from those with very slow growth and long doubling times to highly aggressive lesions with very short doubling times

(Hasegawa et al. 2000; Wang et al. 2000). Thus Hasegawa, in a recent study of mass CT screening, found that tumour volume-doubling times of small peripheral adenocarcinomas ranged from 52 to 1733 days. Such results suggest that overdiagnosis could be an important factor in lung cancer screening with spiral CT and further information on the natural history and behaviour of screen-detected cancers is awaited.

Results of trials of low-dose spiral CT screening for lung cancer in Japan and the USA, which have been conducted in high-risk groups of individuals, have demonstrated that small peripheral lung cancers can be detected in up to 1–2.7% of the screened population and that low-dose spiral CT is significantly more sensitive than chest radiography (Kaneko et al. 1996; Sone et al. 1998; Henschke et al. 1999; Diederich et al. 2000). The Early Lung Cancer Action Project (ELCAP) Study from New York has stimulated most interest. In this study 233 non-calcified nodules were detected in 1000 individuals aged 60 years and over, with a history of at least 10 pack-years of cigarette smoking; 27 lung cancers were detected, of which 23 (81%) were stage I at diagnosis. All patients underwent chest radiography, which proved to be remarkably inferior because only 7 (0.7%) lung cancers were detected on chest radiographs. No cancers were detected on chest radiographs that were missed on spiral CT. Lung biopsy of suspicious nodules was undertaken in 28 of the 233 patients with lung cancer and no patient underwent thoracotomy who did not have lung cancer. These results therefore suggest that low-dose spiral CT not only is sensitive for the detection of peripheral lung cancers but, with follow-up investigation to assess whether the lesion has grown, can also be specific. Follow-up spiral CT at 1 year revealed an incidence rate for nodules of 4% and an incidence rate for new cancers of 1%. Another current trial, the New Mayo Lung Project, funded by the NCI, has screened over 1500 individuals with low-dose spiral CT (Patz et al. 2000). The early results from this project have revealed lung cancer in 1% of the 1250 individuals screened, of whom 60% had stage I disease.

In Japan, studies of lung cancer screening in the 1990s were set up to determine the feasibility of mass screening with spiral CT. These studies, with the subsequent US studies, showed that most (over 80%) cases were stage I at diagnosis (Kaneko et al. 1996; Sone et al. 1998).

The results of these early non-randomised studies of low-dose spiral CT provide the basis for launching RCTs to address the primary issue of whether lung cancer screening can reduce lung cancer mortality.

A question regarding the design of randomised trials using low-dose spiral CT is whether to use chest radiography in the control group. As the value, if any, of chest radiography is currently unknown, there is a strong argument against including it in the control group. Furthermore, in many countries standard practice for the diagnosis of lung cancer is no screening and therefore a trial of low-dose spiral CT against no screening should be regarded as standard. Proponents for using chest radiography in a control group consider that the results of the PLCO study will permit retrospective interpretation of trials of spiral CT versus chest radiography at a future date. On this basis, if chest radiography were shown to be of no value, the control group undergoing chest radiography could be assumed to be similar to a 'no-screen' group. However, it is probably unwise to 'second guess' the results of the PLCO study – there may be an uncertain result, as with the earlier trials, and then the results of a spiral CT trial with chest radiograph screening in the control group would be uninterpretable.

Proposals for lung cancer screening in the UK
LUCAS Trial

The initiative to develop proposals to undertake a trial of low-dose spiral CT in the UK has been led by the Lung Group of the National Cancer Research Institute (NCRI; formerly the UKCCCR). The protocol has been developed by a multidisciplinary group and an application submitted to the Medical Research Council for funding.

The primary research objective of the LUCAS (**lu**ng **ca**ncer **s**creening) Trial is to determine whether lung cancer screening using low-dose spiral CT reduces mortality from lung cancer. A randomised trial of low-dose spiral CT versus no screening in people aged 60 years and over who are smokers is proposed, with lung cancer mortality as the primary endpoint. Smoking cessation advice will be offered to both the screened and the unscreened groups. To determine the feasibility, compliance and probable costs of a large randomised trial, an initial pilot study of 2000 individuals is planned. If this is successful, a full trial of approximately 40 000 individuals will be conducted which, over a 5-year period, is designed to be able to demonstrate a reduction in lung cancer mortality of 25% with a statistical power of 84% at a 5% level of statistical significance. Figure 1.1 is a flow diagram that summarises the study design. In the full trial a cost–benefit analysis will be performed, taking into account the effect of screening, if any, in reducing lung cancer mortality and morbidity, as well as the cost savings made by avoiding treatment of advanced disease. Such data would provide essential information on the costs and benefits of implementing a national lung cancer screening programme in the UK.

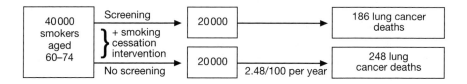

Figure 1.1 Summary of the LUCAS Trial design: screening assuming a 25% reduction in lung cancer mortality as a result of screening and treatment.

Evaluation of pulmonary nodules

Screening studies of low-dose spiral CT have revealed that a large number of indeterminate non-calcified pulmonary nodules are detected, of which only a small proportion prove to be malignant. These non-calcified nodules range in size from only a few millimetres to over a centimetre in diameter. Nodules < 1 cm in diameter are usually impossible to characterise on CT, and biopsy of all such nodules is frequently impractical and undesirable. A strategy for evaluating these non-calcified nodules detected on screening is therefore required. In the UK proposals, we have developed a classification for pulmonary nodules, which is based on the ELCAP Study protocol (Table 1.1). The algorithm for assessing nodules in the UK trial is shown in Figure 1.2.

Table 1.1 Definition and classification of nodules

Category 1	Benign nodules: lesions showing central, rim, uniform or other benign distribution of calcification; fat attenuation within the nodule, clear linear or linear branching densities; known to be stable size for at least 12 months
Category 2	Micronodules, i.e. < 4 mm diameter
Category 3	Indeterminate nodules, 5–10 mm diameter, with undetermined growth rate
Category 4	Nodules > 10 mm diameter not classified as benign, or nodules < 10 mm known to be enlarging on serial CT studies
	Nodule characteristics may include round or spiculated margins, and cavitation. Focal areas of ground glass also included in this category.

A pulmonary nodule is defined as soft-tissue or ground-glass opacity of rounded shape.

Although nodules < 5 mm in diameter would simply be followed by annual screening and nodules > 1 cm in diameter, with morphological features suggestive of malignancy, would be investigated immediately, indeterminate 5- to 10-mm nodules would require intermediate action. Such nodules could be assessed for growth on a 3-monthly high-resolution CT (HRCT) scan through the lesion. Determination of volumetric growth rates using three-dimensional construction computer software has been developed by the ELCAP group (Reeves et al. 2000). Early reports of the use of this software suggest that it is likely to be more accurate than simple bi-dimensional calliper measurements and will reduce the number of false-positive examinations. Based on the average tumour volume-doubling times of non-small cell lung cancers of between 2 and 27 months, the watch-and-wait policy for nodules between 5 and 10 mm in diameter is considered acceptable (Geddes 1979; Usuda et

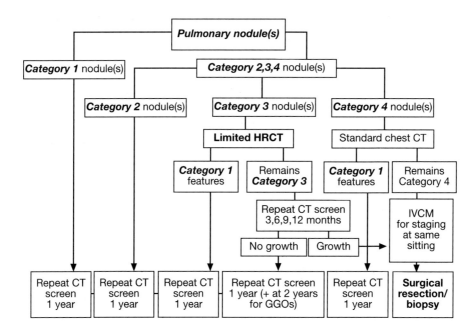

Figure 1.2 Algorithm for assessing pulmonary nodules in the UK LUCAS Trial. GGO, ground-glass opacities; HRCT, high-resolution computed tomography; IVCM, intravenous contrast medium.

al. 1994; Hasegawa et al. 2000; Wang et al. 2000), e.g. a 4-mm lung cancer detected on the prevalence screen and only followed up 1 year later would have a maximum diameter of ≤ 10 mm, provided the tumour volume-doubling time was at least 3 months (P Armstrong, personal communication).

The morphological characteristics of peripheral lung cancers detected on spiral CT range from soft tissue nodules to lesions of ground-glass attenuation. Such ground-glass opacities may be uniform or may show a complex pattern of soft-tissue elements as well as ground-glass elements. Histopathologically, these lesions represent different histologies, ranging from benign lesions through to aggressive adenocarcinomas. Bronchioalveolar adenocarcinomas are of interest because they represent lesions that are unlikely to be identified on chest radiography and may demonstrate a very slow growth pattern (Yang et al. 2001).

Possible hazards of lung cancer screening

Low-dose spiral CT produces good quality CT examinations at a radiation dose of approximately one-sixth that of a conventional CT examination of the chest. This is likely to be less than 2.5 mSv per scan irrespective of the type of scanner used. Adopting the same protocol as Henschke et al. (1999), the patient dose is of the order of 1 mSv (ImPACT CT Scanner Comparison Report). This compares favourably with the average annual environmental exposure of 2.2 mSv in the UK and does not pose a problem. However, it is prudent that the radiation dose of low-dose spiral CT is monitored in a quality control programme in any trials undertaken to evaluate lung cancer screening. In the UK LUCAS Pilot Trial, a mobile scanner will be used. This will have the important advantage of a closely monitored quality control programme in relation to X-ray dose, image quality and adherence to protocol.

Hazards from lung cancer screening also pertain to those resulting from biopsy, thoracotomy and misdiagnosis. Screening is not perfect and individuals entering low-dose spiral CT trials need to be informed about the advantages and disadvantages of screening before recruitment. False-positive spiral CT examinations or false-positive histology/cytology results from biopsy may lead to unnecessary lung resection, introducing the risks of morbidity and mortality associated with thoracic surgery. However, in the ELCAP study, no patient with a benign nodule was referred for thoracotomy. Adoption of a protocol to determine nodule growth before resection or biopsy should minimise this problem. Small peripheral lung cancers may be missed on the initial spiral CT examination, although identified on a subsequent scan. Kakinuma et al. (1999) reported that 7 of 22 lung cancers were missed on initial screening with low-dose spiral CT but, when detected at follow-up, 6 of these were stage I. It should of course be remembered that lung cancers arising in the central airways are likely to be missed on low-dose spiral CT because the technique is insensitive for detecting endobronchial lesions.

The future

Lung cancer screening using low-dose spiral CT is an exciting new approach, which may prove to be worthwhile. If the LUCAS Trial is funded and lung cancer mortality in the UK shown to be reduced by lung cancer screening with low-dose spiral CT, the introduction of a national screening programme would become a practical proposition. This would incur significant capital costs, which would need to be offset against the benefits of screening and of treating symptomatic patients with advanced disease. Dedicated screening centres would be necessary because radiology departments throughout the country would be unable to cope with the enormous increased workload within routine clinical practice. The use of a mobile CT scanner in the LUCAS Pilot Trial will mimic the facilities of a dedicated screening centre, and this too would provide valuable information on the logistics of setting up a national screening service.

Lung cancer screening using spiral CT presents great logistical, radiological, clinical and economic challenges. Interpretation of lung cancer screening CT examinations may be difficult and time-consuming, and if screening were to be introduced on a national basis this would have important radiological workload implications. Skill-mix initiatives and the introduction of computer-aided detection

(CAD) software, which is currently under clinical development, may overcome some of these problems in the longer term. In the short term, the LUCAS Trial would explore these practical issues and endeavour to determine appropriate solutions.

In conclusion, there is now considerable evidence from non-randomised trials that lung cancer screening using low-dose spiral CT can identify small peripheral lung cancers at an early stage of development in asymptomatic patients. Hence, there is now a compelling need to undertake appropriately designed randomised trials to determine whether the detection of early stage peripheral lung cancers will reduce lung cancer mortality and, if so, the magnitude of this reduction. Based on these results it would then be possible to estimate the full costs of screening and to determine whether a national lung cancer screening programme within the UK would be worthwhile.

Acknowledgements

We most gratefully acknowledge the work of our co-applicants of the LUCAS Trial as well as the work of the lead investigators in the participating centres: Dr Martin Muers, Professor Peter Armstrong, Professor John Field, Dr Michael Peake, Professor Elaine Rankin, Dr Richard Neal and Professor Ian Smith (Chairman, NCRI Lung Group).

References

Berrino F, Sant M, Verdecchia A et al. (eds) (1995) *Survival of Cancer Patients in Europe: the EUROCARE Study.* IARC Scientific Publications No. 132. Lyon: International Agency for Research on Cancer.

Brett GZ (1968) The value of lung cancer detection by six-monthly chest radiographs. *Thorax* **23**: 414–420.

CRC Cancerstats (1999) *Mortality – UK,* July. London: Cancer Research Council.

Diederich S, Wormanns D, Lenzen H et al. (2000) Screening for asymptomatic early bronchogenic carcinoma with low dose CT of the chest. *Cancer* **89**: 2483–2484.

Doll R, Peto R, Wheatley K et al. (1994). Mortality in relation to smoking: 40 years' observation on male British doctors. *British Medical Journal* **309**: 901–911.

Flehinger BJ, Melamed MR, Zaman MB et al. (1984) Early lung cancer detection: results of the initial (prevalence) radiologic and cytologic screening in the Memorial Sloan-Kettering study. *American Review of Respiratory Disease* **130**: 555–560.

Fontana RS, Sanderson DR, Woolner LB et al. (1986) Lung cancer screening: the Mayo program. *Journal of Occupational Medicine* **28**: 746–750.

Geddes DM (1979) The natural history of lung cancer: a review based on rates of tumour growth. *British Journal of Diseases of the Chest* **73**: 1–17.

Gohagan JK, Prorok JC, Kramer BS et al. (1995) The prostate, lung, colorectal and ovarian screening trial of the National Cancer Institute. *Cancer* **75**: 1869–1873.

Hasegawa M, Sone S, Takashima S et al. (2000) Growth rate of small lung cancers detected on mass CT screening. *British Journal of Radiology* **73**: 1252–1259.

Henschke CI, McCauley DI, Yankelevitz DF et al. (1999) Early Lung Cancer Action Project: overall design and findings from baseline screening. *The Lancet* **354**: 99–105.

ImPACT CT Scanner Comparison Report Issue 12 MDA/00/11.

Kakinuma R, Ohmatsu H, Kaneko M et al. (1999) Detection failures in spiral CT for screening for lung cancer: analysis of CT findings. *Radiology* **212**: 61–66.

Kaneko M, Eguchi K, Ohmatsu H et al. (1996) Peripheral lung cancer: screening and detection with low-dose spiral CT versus radiography. *Radiology* **201**: 798–802.

Kubik A, Parkin DM, Khlat M et al. (1990) Lack of benefit from semi-annual screening for cancer of the lung: follow-up report of a randomized controlled trial on a population of high-risk males in Czechoslovakia. *International Journal of Cancer* **45**: 26–33.

Kubik AK, Parkin DM, Zatloukal P (2000) Czech study on lung cancer screening: post-trial follow-up of lung cancer deaths up to year 15 since enrollment. *Cancer* **89**: 2363–2368.

Lopez A (1995) The lung cancer epidemic in developed countries. In: Lopez AD, Caselli G, Valkonen T (eds), *Adult Mortality in Developed Countries: From description to explanation.* Oxford University Press, pp. 111–113.

Martini N, Bains MS, Burt ME (1995) Incidence of local recurrence and second primary tumors in resected stage I lung cancer. *Journal of Thoracic and Cardiovascular Surgery* **109**: 120–129.

Mountain CF (1977) Assessment of the role of surgery for control of lung cancer. *Annals of Thoracic Surgery* **24**: 365–373.

Nash FA, Morgan JM, Tomkins JG (1968) South London Lung Cancer Study. *British Medical Journal* **ii**: 715–721.

Nesbitt JC, Putnam JC Jr, Walsh GL et al. (1995) Survival in early-stage non small cell lung cancer. *Annals of Thoracic Surgery* **60**: 466–472.

Patz EF Jr, Goodman PC, Bepler G (2000) Screening for lung cancer. *New England Journal of Medicine* **343**: 1627–1633.

Reeves AP, Kostis WJ (2000) Computer-aided diagnosis of small pulmonary nodules. *Seminars in Ultrasound, CT and MRI* **21**: 116–128.

Shah R, Sabanathan S, Richardson J et al. (1996) Results of surgical treatment of stage I and II lung cancer. *Journal of Cardiovascular Surgery* **37**: 169–172.

Sone S, Takashima S, Li F et al. (1998) Mass screening for lung cancer with mobile spiral computed tomography scanner. *The Lancet* **351**: 1242–1245.

Tockman MS (1986) Survival and mortality from lung cancer in a screened population: the John Hopkins Study. *Chest* **89**: 324–325S.

Usuda K, Saito Y, Sagawa M et al. (1994) Tumor doubling time and prognostic assessment of patients with primary lung cancer. *Cancer* **74**: 2239–2244.

Wang JC, Sone S, Feng L et al. (2000) Rapidly growing small peripheral lung cancers detected by screening CT: correlation between radiological appearance and pathological features. *British Journal of Radiology* **73**: 930–937.

Wilde J (1989) A 10-year follow-up of semi-annual screening for early detection of lung cancer in the Erfurt Country, GDR. *European Respiratory Journal* **2**: 656–662.

Yang Z-G, Sone S, Li F et al. (2001) Visibility of small peripheral lung cancers on chest radiographs: influence of densitometric parameters, CT values and tumour type. *British Journal of Radiology* **74**: 32–41.

PART 2

Surgical intervention

Chapter 2

Downstaging disease before surgery: a review of current strategies

Peter Goldstraw

Introduction

The definition of 'downstaging' employed for this chapter is any manoeuvre, statistical or therapeutic, designed to reduce the *perceived* extent of disease, as assessed by the TNM stage, before definitive treatment. Although this chapter focuses on lung cancer, and non-small cell lung cancer (NSCLC) in particular, and the definitive treatment is surgery, some of the principles apply more generally. The emphasis on 'perceived' in this definition is to remind us all that the clinical/ evaluative stage (cTNM) on which we base our treatment decisions is inaccurate and fallible for a number of reasons.

First, there is no standard staging protocol and the evaluation of the case will be influenced by the availability of staging investigations. Although computed tomography (CT) scanners should be available at all cancer units, there will be variations in the speed of the scanner and the protocol used. If the physician has undertaken a CT of the chest during the diagnostic work-up, he or she may be reluctant to send the patient back for a staging CT of the abdomen if this entails further delay or a trip to another hospital. Instead abdominal ultrasonography may be performed locally with less delay. Although, in the best hands, this has the same sensitivity and specificity as CT it is operator dependent and rarely validated. Positron emission tomography (PET) is available only in a few centres (London, Manchester, Cambridge, Aberdeen), and even here few units have sufficient access to use it routinely. Only an experienced thoracic surgeon can perform mediastinoscopy. The physician may therefore be tempted into assessing the pathological status of mediastinal lymph nodes on the basis of their size on CT, a notoriously unreliable technique, if access to such a surgeon is difficult or will create further delays. This is understandable given that the evolving guidelines on cancer care for the present place greater emphasis on speed than quality outcome measurements.

Second, the interpretation of each staging investigation is also, to some extent, subjective and will be influenced by the physician's overall assessment of the patient. If the patient is slightly frail and clearly anxious by the prospect of surgery, the radiologist's report of 'borderline' mediastinal nodes and a 'bulky' adrenal gland may more readily be interpreted as N2 and M1 disease. Such an approach may well be in the patient's best interest although resulting in less accurate staging. It is difficult to quantify these factors, although we all recognise that it occurs, and surgeons in particular see patients who have questioned such decisions and are shown, on more detailed staging, to be operable. One prospective, multicentre study (Lopez-Encuentra et al. 2002) has shown that central revision of cTNM by a review board applying rigorous definitions of stage and other criteria results in considerable downstaging of the intrathoracic disease. In this study cT stage was reduced in 11% of cases and only upstaged in 1%, whereas cN stage was reduced in 18% of cases and upstaged in none.

One of our studies has shown that even the most rigorous cTNM stage will prove inaccurate in over half of all cases when patients are subjected to detailed intrathoracic staging at thoracotomy (Fernando and Goldstraw 1990). In this study cT was downstaged in 3% and upstaged in 16% of cases whereas cN was downstaged in 7% and upstaged in 38%. The net result was that cTN was inaccurate in 53% of all cases.

These contrary influences may cancel themselves out, but this is uncertain. Clearly any assessment of cTNM that leads to treatment other than thoracotomy will be open to considerable error. In addition, if 'effective' therapy is applied before thoracotomy our understanding of the original extent of the disease will always be less than perfect. With these cautions, let us look at the options for downstaging and the probable benefits of such an approach.

Discussion

Induction therapy

Additional treatment before surgery is now better known as 'induction' therapy. Radiotherapy was the first modality used and is still popular for the tiny minority of patients with Pancoast's tumours who are being considered for resection (Paulson 1975). It will shrink tumours, but this may have little influence on the ease of resection and none at all on the feasibility of complete resection. A tumour may be irresectable by reason of invasion at one margin, such as invasion into the vertebral body or other important mediastinal structures. It is this edge of the tumour that is most likely to be missed by the radiation field and, even when CT planning is used, there may be perfectly reasonable considerations that cause the radiation oncologist to reduce the radiation dose at this point, such as concerns for the spinal cord or oesophagus. Induction radiotherapy adds to the morbidity of subsequent resection and is therefore unpopular with surgeons. There is no proof of its value.

Relapse patterns after resection of NSCLC (Feld et al. 1984) clearly show that cure is most frequently frustrated by the appearance of metastatic disease that was occult at the time of surgery. The use of chemotherapy as an induction agent has therefore received most attention.

Chemoradiation has been shown to result in the highest pathological response rate but is also associated with greater toxicity and operative morbidity (Vansteenkiste et al. 1998a).

The literature on induction therapy has been further confused by a failure to specify the intention of such treatment in individual studies. The word "downstaging" may be used in several ways. First, downstaging has been used in an attempt to render irresectable disease resectable. There are anecdotal reports suggesting that this may prove feasible. However, as there is no clear definition of irresectability before exploratory thoracotomy and no studies using 'second-look' thoracotomy, this role for induction therapy has had to be assessed from studies in patients who are considered to be 'marginally' resectable. It is impossible to know in such uncontrolled studies whether there has been an increase in the number of cases that were shown subsequently to be resectable (Rusch et al. 1993). How does one decide which 'marginally' resectable cases have improved sufficiently to justify an attempt at resection? There are additional concerns as to the survival advantage achieved by the resection of such 'marginal' cases when compared with the results using advanced radiation techniques such as continuous hyperfractionated accelerated radiotherapy (CHART) and present chemoradiation protocols. Overall, it seems unlikely that the use of induction therapy in such cases will result in any significant increase in the proportion of sufferers undergoing worthwhile surgery.

Second, we may downstage in an attempt to render medically inoperable cases operable. Such cases are by definition thought to be resectable, but the patient is insufficiently robust to tolerate the probable extent of resection. Again, there are no randomised studies and any benefit is likely to prove minimal. If resection proves feasible and safe, was this a result of downstaging? Was the resection of less lung parenchyma made possible by more imaginative techniques such as bronchoplasty or angioplasty? Is the resection of less lung parenchyma after induction therapy likely to result in cure or are we leaving microscopic viable malignancy *in situ* to frustrate our attempts at cure?

Last, and most commonly, "downstaging" treatment has been used in an attempt to render oncologically inoperable disease operable. In such cases the disease is considered resectable but the results do not justify the mortality and morbidity of surgery when compared with other methods of treatment. This situation is most usually associated with N2 disease that has been detected, and sometimes histologically confirmed, before thoracotomy. Such disease not only reduces the prospect of complete resection but, more importantly, is associated with high relapse rates caused by occult micrometastatic disease. Clearly, the protocols used in this situation must use chemotherapy for its systemic effects but experience with chemotherapy in limited disease SCLC, a more responsive tumour, is not encouraging. Survival in this disease is poor and usually decided by the appearance of metastatic deposits (Souhami and Law 1990). After induction chemotherapy, do we choose only to operate on patients who show a radiographic response – using this as a surrogate marker for the effect of chemotherapy at the presumed metastatic sites? There is a poor correlation between radiographic responses and the pathological effects achieved with chemotherapy at the primary site and in any nodal deposits.

The changes in PET activity after induction chemotherapy may prove to be a better tool to select those patients who should go on to thoracotomy (Vansteenkiste et al. 1998b).

Randomised trials

Of the few randomised studies of induction chemotherapy, two of the best studied the role of induction chemotherapy in N2 disease. Although the studies by Rosell et al. (1994) and Roth et al. (1994) seem similar, using induction chemotherapy before thoracotomy in one arm and surgery alone in the other arm, the results offer differing interpretations. Both studies enrolled stage IIIA cases and, although terminated for valid statistical reasons, were subsequently too small to compensate for the heterogeneous nature of the study population. In addition both made extensive use of postoperative radiotherapy, 60 Gy for all cases in the Rosell study and 60–66 Gy in over half of each arm in the Roth study. In the Rosell study, there was a statistically significant benefit to chemotherapy, with a median survival of 26 months compared with 8 months in the surgery-alone arm ($p = 0.001$). One has to ask whether, with such modest survival, either arm benefited from surgery, and whether one should conclude that, in this population, the study merely showed that these IIIA (N2) inoperable cases chemoradiotherapy proved more effective than radiotherapy alone. In the Roth study, there was a statistically significant survival benefit in the chemotherapy arm. This remained also on subsequent follow-up (Roth et al. 1998), although the level of significance fell. Median survival was reported to be 21 months in the chemotherapy and surgery arm compared with 14 months in the surgery-alone arm. The 5-year survival rate was also superior in the chemotherapy and surgery arm: 36% versus 15%. Selection in this study was clearly more discriminating and only half of the suitable cases were enrolled into the study, more extensive use being made of mediastinoscopy to exclude N3 disease and irresectable N2 cases. Surgeons have shown in several series that long-term survival can be achieved with a small subset of N2 cases (Martini and Flehinger 1987; Naruke et al. 1988; Goldstraw et al. 1994) and this study probably shows a survival benefit for chemotherapy in such cases. The question remains as to the benefit of surgery in such cases when compared with newer radiation and chemoradiation protocols.

The most interesting question to be asked of induction chemotherapy relates to its role in operable disease. Even in stage I disease, the results of resection do not meet the expectations of our patients, and only 55% achieve long-term survival (Mountain 1997). There are practical and theoretical reasons why induction chemotherapy should be studied in this setting (Johnson and Piantadosi 1994). Chemotherapy should prove more effective against the smaller volume disease usually found in operable cases. There should be fewer drug-resistant cells and better penetration of the drugs before surgical manipulation. The target dose will be achieved in a higher proportion of patients in a preoperative setting in which patients have not incurred the morbidity, temporary or permanent, consequent upon operation. Response can be objectively assessed and postoperative regimens used selectively. A larger population would be recruited into such trials such that the value of induction therapy can be properly assessed. We conducted a pilot study with our colleagues at the Royal Marsden Hospital to study the feasibility of such therapy in all operable cases (de Boer et al. 1999). It showed that such treatment was well tolerated. We did not find that the delay before surgery resulted in progression or that toxicity concerns prevented subsequent operation. However, others have suggested that resection may prove more hazardous and acute lung injury (ALI), already the greatest cause of postoperative deaths (Kutlu et al. 2000), may be more common after induction chemotherapy (Fowler et al. 1993). Recruitment to our study proved difficult and this has dogged the subsequent randomised trial conducted by the MRC (LU22). If induction chemotherapy is to be effective it is in this role that it should show a survival advantage, but the question remains unanswered.

Conclusions

The value of induction therapy in NSCLC remains unproven and its use should be restricted to prospective, randomised studies. If it is shown to be of value, there will be enormous resource implications for our national cancer strategy. It remains to be shown whether the prognosis of any group of patients is improved by such treatment and whether such treatment is cost-effective.

Recommendations

The priorities for our National Cancer Strategy should be:

- To focus on tobacco control and smoking cessation.
- To strive to reduce the delays in patient presentation and evaluation. In a recent study the cumulative delay between the onset of symptoms and referral to a surgeon with a diagnosis of lung cancer was 3.5 times the subsequent delay until surgical treatment (Lee et al., in press).
- To improve access to dedicated thoracic surgeons, so that those patients who are operable by conventional criteria undergo surgery. There is a national shortage of such surgeons in the UK and too many operations are undertaken by surgeons without the experience or training to evaluate such cases properly, or who are unfamiliar with the lung-sparing techniques that have been shown to reduce morbidity and mortality without compromising survival. The shortage of such expertise may undermine the value of multidisciplinary meetings and forcing physicians to make the decisions regarding operability without sufficient surgical input. Steps taken by the Specialist Advisory Committee in Cardiothoracic Surgery in the UK will address this problem over time.

References

de Boer RH, Smith IE, Pastorino U et al. (1999) Pre-operative chemotherapy in early stage resectable non-small-cell lung cancer: a randomized feasibility study justifying a multicentre phase III trial. *British Journal of Cancer* **79**: 1514–1518.

Feld R, Rubinstein LV, Weisenburger TH (1984) Sites of recurrence in resected stage I non-small-cell lung cancer: A guide for future studies. *Journal of Clinical Oncology* **2**: 1352–1358.

Fernando HC, Goldstraw P (1990) The accuracy of clinical evaluative intrathoracic staging in lung cancer as assessed by postsurgical pathologic staging. *Cancer* **65**: 2503–2506.

Fowler WC, Langer CJ, Curran WJ (1993) Postoperative complications after combined neoadjuvant treatment of lung cancer. *Annals of Thoracic Surgery* **55**: 986–989.

Goldstraw P, Mannam GC, Kaplan DK, Michail P (1994) Surgical management of non-small-cell lung cancer with ipsilateral mediastinal node metastasis (N2 disease). *Journal of Thoracic and Cardiovascular Surgery* **107**: 19–27.

Johnson DH, Piantadosi S (1994) Chemotherapy for resectable stage III non-small-cell lung cancer – can that dog hunt? *Journal of the National Cancer Institute* **86**: 650–651.

Kutlu CA, Williams EA, Evans TW, Pastorino U, Goldstraw P (2000) Acute lung injury and acute respiratory distress syndrome after pulmonary resection. *Annals of Thoracic Surgery* **69**: 376–380.

Lee J, Marchbank A, Goldstraw P (2002) Implementation of the British Thoracic Society recommendations for organising the care of patients with lung cancer: the surgeon's perspective. *Annals of The Royal College of Surgeons of England (London)* **84**: in press.

Lopez-Encuentra A, de la Camara AG, Bronchogenic Carcinoma Cooperative Group of the Spanish Society of Pneumology and Thoracic Surgery (2002) The validation of a central review board of staging prior to surgery for non-small-cell lung cancer: impact on prognosis. A multicenter study. *Respiration* in press.

Martini N, Flehinger BJ (1987) The role of surgery in N2 lung cancer. *Surgical Clinics of North America* **67**: 1037–1049.

Mountain CF (1997) Revisions in the International System for Staging Lung Cancer. *Chest* **111**: 1710–1717.

Naruke T, Goya T, Tsuchiya R, Suemasu K (1988) The importance of surgery to non-small cell carcinoma of lung with mediastinal lymph node metastasis. *Annals of Thoracic Surgery* **46**: 603–610.

Paulson DL (1975) Carcinomas in the superior pulmonary sulcus. *Journal of Thoracic and Cardiovascular Surgery* **70**: 1095–1104.

Rosell R, Gomez-Codina J, Camps C et al. (1994) A randomized trial comparing preoperative chemotherapy plus surgery with surgery alone in patients with non-small-cell lung cancer. *New England Journal of Medicine* **330**: 153–158.

Roth JA, Fossella F, Komaki R et al. (1994) A randomized trial comparing perioperative chemotherapy and surgery with surgery alone in resectable stage IIIA non-small-cell lung cancer. *Journal of the National Cancer Institute* **86**: 673–680.

Roth JA, Atkinson EN, Fossella F et al. (1998) Long-term follow-up of patients enrolled in a randomised trial comparing perioperative chemotherapy and surgery with surgery alone in resectable stage IIIA non-small-cell lung cancer. *Lung Cancer* **21**: 1–6.

Rusch VW, Albain KS, Crowley JJ et al. (1993) Surgical resection of stage IIIA and IIIB non-small-cell lung cancer after concurrent induction chemoradiotherapy: A Southwest Oncology Group trial. *Journal of Thoracic and Cardiovascular Surgery* **105**: 97–106.

Souhami RL, Law K (1990) Longevity in small cell lung cancer. A report to the Lung Cancer Subcommittee of the United Kingdom Coordinating Committee for Cancer Research. *British Journal of Cancer* **61**: 584–589.

Vansteenkiste J, De Leyn P, Deneffe G et al. (1998a) Present status of induction treatment in stage IIIA-N2 non-small cell lung cancer: a review. *European Journal of Cardio-thoracic Surgery* **13**: 1–12.

Vansteenkiste J, Stroobants SG, De Leyn P, Dupont PJ, Verbeken E, The Leuvan Lung Cancer Group (1998b) Potential use of FDG-PET scan after induction chemotherapy in surgically staged IIIa-N2 non-small-cell lung cancer: a prospective pilot study. *Annals of Oncology* **9**: 1193–1198.

Chapter 3

Extended resection and reconstructive surgery: a review of current strategies

Francis Wells

The surgical resection rates for lung cancer in the UK remain among the lowest in Europe. Other healthcare systems achieve a resection rate of up to or just over 20%. In Britain today, the national average for most centres is under 10%. This unsatisfactory resection rate can be used as a "barometer" of care for patients with lung cancer. Not only does this fact point out the severe shortfall in services in this country, but also the needed potential in exploring surgical resection of more locally advanced tumours. Those countries with resection rates that are routinely in excess of 20% have centres that are actively engaged in down-staging chemotherapy trials and extended resections in a controlled and carefully observed environment. It is difficult to develop the more advanced surgical techniques in a constrained system.

The most important development in the surgical management of lung cancer has been the widespread introduction of tumour staging. Full prospective and retrospective post-surgical pathological staging of the tumour, in all patients, is vital if the results of extended resections are to be understood in the future. Spread of the tumour to the mediastinal lymph nodes and beyond portends a short survival time. Therefore, it is argued that the pain and risk that a patient experiences with major surgery are not justified if the chance of extended survival or cure is not significantly increased.

As data have accumulated, the understanding of the implications of mediastinal lymph node involvement has become more sophisticated. Although involvement of paratracheal and subcarinal nodes means a 5-year survival rate of less than 5% in most series, para-aortic and aortopulmonary window nodes seem to fare somewhat better (up to 25% in some series).

Direct mediastinal and chest wall invasion have also been viewed with pessimism by many physicians. However, in the absence of mediastinal lymph node involvement (groups 7, 10 and 4 particularly), selected cases can achieve worthwhile mid- and long-term survival.

In addition, although most patients with advanced local disease fare poorly, many surgeons have observed long-term survival in occasional patients with extended resection for locally advanced disease, especially in the absence of lymph node involvement. All of these observations have led to a rethink about the role of extended resection for patients with lung cancer.

In this chapter the author wishes to explore some of the possibilities for extended resection and to consider the scientific boundaries that restrict the cure rate for patients with lung cancer.

Lung cancer like breast cancer is frequently a disseminated disease at presentation. Of patients with the disease, 70–80% will have inoperable disease when first seen. This is as a result of blood-borne and lymphatic spread distant from the primary site. However, if local spread is restricted to areas that can be included within the resection, why should we not be able to expect a chance of cure? The best hope for cure still rests with surgical extirpation of the cancer.

A real concern of attending physicians and surgeons, however, is that if the use of surgery is too liberal then a significant number of patients will be subjected to unnecessary operations and the trauma that this entails.

What does extended resection mean?

Extended resection means the resection of a tumour beyond the readily accepted guidelines for staged tumours. This includes the following:

- Chest wall and diaphragmatic extension
- Superior sulcus tumours
- Involvement of the heart and/or the great vessels
- Bronchoplastic resections such as carina and main trachea
- Complete lymph node clearance within the hemi-thorax.

Some surgeons would include those patients who have other complicating factors such as advanced emphysema or coronary artery disease.

In patients with emphysema, the effect of the removal of a lobe that is badly affected by the disease may equate to the beneficial effects attributable to surgery for lung volume reduction. Hence a patient who was previously deemed to be inoperable might, with the application of that kind of lateral thought, be brought into the operable category. Similarly patients with coronary artery disease may be considered inoperable because of the extent of the coronary lesions. However, re-vascularising the heart may well render the patient operable.

Using the TNM classification, all stage I (T1N0 and T2N0) and stage II (T1N1, T2N1 and T3N0) tumours are regarded as operable. Stage IIIA (T3N1M0, T1N2M0, T2N2M0 and T3N2M0) and IIIB (T4N0 and T4N1) have not been regarded as operable by all surgical oncologists.

A T3 tumour is one of any size that directly invades the chest wall, superior sulcus, diaphragm, mediastinal pleura, parietal pericardium and main bronchus within 2 cm of the carina or with associated pulmonary collapse.

A T4 tumour is one of any size that invades the mediastinum or contents, vertebrae or carina, or has an associated pleuro-pericardial effusion of malignant origin. The presence of satellite lesions in the ipsilateral lung also falls within this category.

Identification of real mediastinal invasion preoperatively remains a significant problem. Subtle degrees of invasion or mere inflammatory adhesion of the tumour to the mediastinum is not possible to diagnose reliably on either computed tomography (CT) or magnetic resonance imaging (MRI). Often the only way forward is with surgical exploration. Indeed if a unit is not experiencing a failed thoracotomy rate of 2–3% per annum, potentially operable tumours are probably being missed.

In a recently published large study of post-surgical results, Naruke and colleagues (2001) in Tokyo have demonstrated that, in clinical stage IIIA disease, a 22.7% 5-year survival rate can be obtained. This fell to 20.1% for stage IIIB tumours. Interestingly post-surgical pathological restaging increased the survivors in the IIIA group to 23.6%, but reduced the survivors in the IIIB group to 16.5%. Superior sulcus tumours and those invading the diaphragm fared least well.

Chest wall and diaphragm invasion

A peripheral lung cancer invading the parietal pleura or deeper into the chest wall muscle or ribs can be resected very easily. Many of the smaller areas of involvement (up to 5 cm or so), especially when covered by the scapula, can be resected without reconstruction. However, if the area is larger, then the chest wall can be reconstructed using a double layer of polypropylene mesh, sandwiching a methyl methacrylate bone cement plate. This composite can be shaped to match the natural shape of the chest wall.

Similarly, invasion of the diaphragm can be dealt with by local resection and reconstruction using the same plastic mesh in a single layer. Indeed small areas of the right hemi-diaphragm do not need reconstruction at all because of the presence of the liver underneath.

These kind of extended resections have been practised since the earliest development of thoracic surgery and are relatively non-controversial. They should be part of the standard repertoire of the skilled thoracic surgeon.

The most important predictor of outcome in this situation is the presence or absence of mediastinal node invasion. In two publications (Pitz et al. 1996; Elia et al. 2001) from Italy and the Netherlands, respectively, worthwhile survival was achieved for patients with chest wall invasion in the absence of mediastinal node invasion. In both studies the presence of tumour in mediastinal nodes met with poor or no survival. In addition, the Dutch group demonstrated that spillage of tumour into the thorax during resection also resulted in a worse outcome.

Superior sulcus tumours

If tumours arising at the apex of either upper lobe invade the chest wall at an early stage, the brachial plexus, posterior angle of the first rib and/or the vertebral body may be invaded. This will result in severe local pain and referred pain from the particular nerve roots that are affected. Horner's syndrome and pain in the shoulder and arm are common and intractable. The combined use of radiotherapy and local resection has been used for some time. The results are poor for most patients in the mid to long term, but may result in the significant reduction or cessation of symptoms for a worthwhile period.

If the tumour invades within the neck of the first rib and its associated vertebral body, resection is rarely successful. Published results of very extensive local resection have met with improved results in the hands of Dartevelle and associates (1993). However, widespread adoption of these techniques is probably not wise until longer-term results are available.

Mediastinal invasion

The discovery that a tumour is invading the mediastinal structures almost invariably meets with a very nihilistic attitude. Direct spread into the mediastinal fat almost invariably means that the tumour cannot be completely removed and hence surgery should not be undertaken. However, in some circumstances resection is possible. Direct tumour extension into a mediastinal structure that can be removed with a good margin of uninvolved tissue should not deter resection, e.g. if the tumour includes pericardium that can be resected, most surgeons would do so. If the resected area is large, the defect can be repaired with a bovine pericardial patch or synthetic material. Extension into the pulmonary veins up to the left atrial wall can often be removed by extending the resection into the pericardium. Occasionally, direct invasion of the superior vena cava (SVC) can be managed by a local resection and reconstruction, as long as the extent is limited.

A recent paper from France demonstrated that worthwhile survival can be obtained by extended resection in patients with mediastinal invasion, as long as there is no significant mediastinal lymph node involvement (Doddoli et al. 2001). Overall 5-year actuarial survival rate in 29 patients who underwent superior vena caval (SVC) aortic, left atrial and carinal resection was 28% (median 11 months). In addition to the poor prognostic effect of positive nodal disease, incomplete resection was shown to be a disaster with early recurrence and poor mid-term outcome.

In the left side of the chest, extension into the aorta is generally considered to be unresectable, but occasionally very localised involvement can be removed and reconstructed.

The problem with all of these extended resections is that the number of properly reported cases with full staging information is limited as are the follow-up data. Case numbers are generally small and long-term follow-up reports are significantly lacking.

In any of these situations, however, if there is mediastinal lymph nodal involvement, the outlook is very poor and resection should not be undertaken.

Carinal and other bronchoplastic resections

Sleeve resection for upper lobe tumours that arise at the origin of the upper lobe bronchi is a technique that has been around for many years. In the absence of lymph node involvement, it is an excellent way of extending resection for patients with poor lung function. By reconnecting the intermediate bronchus on the left, or lower lobe bronchus on the right, back to the main bronchus, resection of tumours that are otherwise inoperable because of poor functional reserve becomes possible. They are accepted and non-controversial techniques. Surgeons who are not trained in their safe execution do their patients a disservice.

Techniques are available for resection and reconstruction of the carina for local bronchogenic carcinoma extension. These are more controversial because not only are they more difficult to complete safely, but also because there is very little data about them. However, in 1991 Grillo and Mathisen published a small series that demonstrated that the procedure was possible in skilled hands. Even this distinguished group had problems, however. Three early separations of the resected ends occurred and four patients suffered anastosmotic stenosis. There were five absolute survivors at 5 years from an original group of 37 patients, and an actuarial 5-year survival rate of 19%. Clearly, these types of procedures should be concentrated in a few skilled hands and all the data prospectively gathered.

Tumour down-staging

With the advent of modern chemotherapy protocols, there has been a reconsideration of tumours that are deemed to be inoperable as a result of mediastinal invasion. A number of patients seem to experience regression of local mediastinal invasion after completion of chemotherapy. Restaging with repeat CT may demonstrate shrinkage away from the mediastinum. There are now a number of reports of the early outcome following resection in this situation. Although these do hold some promise, there is no robust RCT data or even long-term outcome for this group of patients.

In addition, this kind of approach is not without potential additional risk. There have been a number of reports of increased pulmonary permeability following surgical resection after chemotherapy. In appraising the risk for patients the cumulative risk of both the chemotherapy regimen and the surgery have to be summated.

Conclusions

In carefully selected cases, extended resection for locally advanced disease can be achieved safely in the modern era of thoracic surgery. There are techniques that can be used to solve most of the problems that confront the surgeon. However, as with all things surgical, just because a procedure can be done it does not mean that it should be done. An unnecessary surgical assault on a patient cannot be justified.

The single most important predictor of outcome is the nodal status of the patient. Disease within the mediastinal lymph nodes represents dissemination away from the primary site and local resection alone will not cure the disease.

The effect of adjunctive chemo- and radiotherapy is under investigation, and all of these patients should be managed and studied as part of a properly constructed and well-powered clinical trial.

References

Dartevelle PG, Chapelier AR, Macchiarini P et al. (1993) Anterior thoracic approach for radical resection of lung tumors invading the thoracic inlet. *Journal of Thoracic and Cardiovascular Surgery* **105**: 1025–1034.

Doddoli C, Rollet G, Thomas P et al. (2001) Is lung cancer surgery justified in patients with direct mediastinal invasion? *European Journal of Cardio-thoracic Surgery* **20**: 339–343.

Elia S, Griffo S, Costabile R, Ferrante G (2001) Surgical treatment of lung cancer invading chest wall: a retrospective analysis of 110 patients. *European Journal of Cardio-thoracic Surgery* **20**: 356–360.

Mathisen D, Grillo H (1991) Carinal resection for bronchogenic carcinoma. *Journal of Thoracic and Cardiovascular Surgery* **102**: 16–23.

Naruke T, Tsuchiya R, Kondo H, Asamura H (2001) Prognosis and survival after resection for bronchogenic carcinoma based on the 1997 TNM-staging classification: The Japanese experience. *Annals of Thoracic Surgery* **71**: 1759–1764.

Pitz CC, Brutel de la riviere A, Elbers H, Westermann CJ, van den Bosch MM (1996) Surgical treatment of 125 patients with non-small cell cancer and chest wall involvement. *Thorax* **51**: 846–850.

PART 3

Medical intervention

Chapter 4

CHART, CHARTWEL and combined modalities: evidence for clinical effectiveness and the consequences of under-utilization

Michele I Saunders

Until the 1970s solid tumours were considered to be slowly growing. This was based on the clinically observed time taken for tumours to double their size, which was usually measured in weeks or months (Steele and Buell 1971). The overall duration of a course of radiotherapy, usually no more than 6 or 7 weeks, was therefore considered unlikely to influence the outcome; the total radiation dose seemed a much more important consideration. In the early 1980s research carried out at the Gray Laboratory, Mount Vernon, and at other institutions, showed that many human tumours had the potential to double their cell numbers in a matter of a few days (Bennett et al. 1992); this was called the potential doubling time or T_{pot}. The difference between the volume doubling time and the potential cell doubling time is the result of the death of cells before going on to further division. More than 90% of the progeny of cell division may die in the unperturbed tumour as a result of lack of nutrition or programmed apoptosis. When, however, active treatment is given, whether by chemotherapy or radiotherapy, the natural cell loss may greatly diminish, and the progeny of each cell division may survive and go on to further divisions so that a rapid cellular repopulation takes place. Clinicians may well be happily watching a tumour regressing in bulk but, at the cellular level, rapid proliferation may be taking place, producing cells that will survive the course of treatment. The potential cell doubling time of non-small cell lung cancer is estimated to average 7 days (Wilson et al. 1988) and so many cell doublings could occur during a 6- to 7-week course of radiotherapy. Some radiobiologists and clinicians consider that the cell doubling time may actually accelerate during treatment, making the situation even worse.

Based on this biological research, protocols of radiotherapy were devised which shortened the overall duration of radiotherapy to minimise the opportunity for cellular repopulation; this is called acceleration. One of the most accelerated regimens to be brought into clinical practice is CHART (**c**ontinuous **h**yperfractionated **a**ccelerated **r**adiotherapy) where the overall duration of a course of treatment is reduced from 42 to 12 days. To achieve this, the regimen took into account other radiobiological research then emerging, including evidence to suggest that, by use of many small individual radiation doses (fractions), the incidence of late effects could be reduced (Withers et al. 1982; Thames et al. 1982). The scheme therefore included three small fractions per day (Figure 4.1) with a 6-hour interfraction interval and radiotherapy commenced on a Monday, and was given continuously for 12 days, finishing on the Friday of the following week, so including one weekend. As 1.5 Gy was given per fraction at 8am, 2pm and 8pm, a total dose of 54 Gy was achieved. Pilot studies of CHART in non-small cell carcinoma took place at Mount Vernon between 1990 and 1995, and a significant improvement in survival was revealed when the result was compared with a previously studied group of patients (Saunders and Dische 1990). These findings led the Medical Research Council, Department of Health and Cancer Research Campaign to fund a multicentre randomised controlled trial in which CHART was compared with conventional radiotherapy using 60 Gy given in 6 weeks, using 2 Gy/fraction daily from Monday to Friday.

	Dose per fraction (Gy)	No. of doses	Total dose (Gy)	Overall duration (days)	Interval between treatments of each day (h)	Weeks						
						1	2	3	4	5	6	7
Conventional	2	33	66	45	24	IIIII	IIIII	IIIII	IIIII	IIIII	IIIII	III
CHART	1.5	36	54	12	6	IIIIIII IIIIIII IIIIIII	IIIII IIIII IIIII					
CHARTWEL	1.5	40	60	18	6	IIIII IIIII IIIII	IIIII IIIII IIIII	IIII III III				

Figure 4.1 Conventional, CHART and CHARTWEL: accelerated schedules of radiotherapy that have been used in non-small cell lung cancer.

Thirteen centres in the UK and Europe took part in the study and 563 patients with non-small cell carcinoma were entered between 1990 and 1995. Acute morbidity, mainly oesophagitis, occurred earlier than with conventional radiotherapy and was slightly more troublesome but settled within the same period of time and was thus not an important disadvantage to the regimen. Late radiation morbidity was low, certainly no more than with conventional treatment. At the conclusion of entry to the CHART trial an advantage to CHART was evident (Saunders et al. 1996) and, at 5 years from entry of the last patient, benefit has been maintained in terms of survival, local tumour control, disease-free survival and metastasis-free survival (Saunders et al. 1996, 1997, 1999).

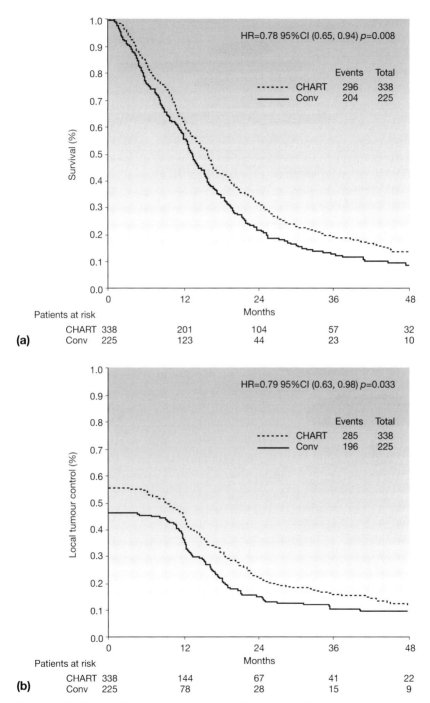

Figure 4.2 Kaplan–Meier curves: (a) overall survival; (b) local tumour control by treatment allocated for all 563 patients randomised.

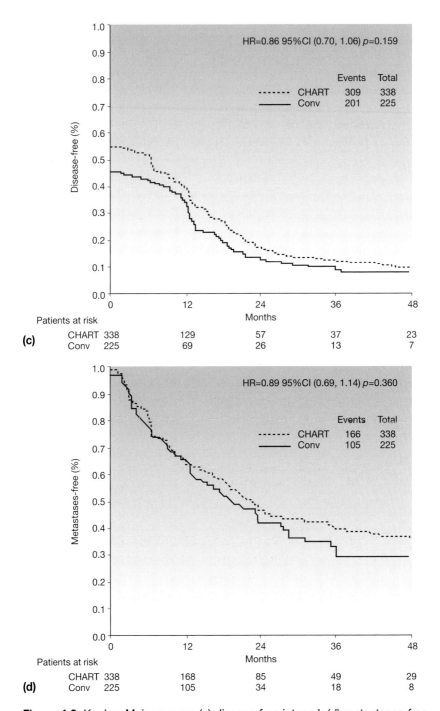

Figure 4.2 Kaplan–Meier curves: (c) disease-free interval; (d) metastases-free interval by treatment allocated for all 563 patients randomised.

An international comparison of the result of CHART was achieved by comparing the results with those published of the meta-analysis of chemotherapy added to conventional radiotherapy in the treatment of non-small cell lung cancer. The meta-analysis revealed that those trials in which *cis*-platinum was used were the only ones that gave benefit, and these gave a 4% improvement in overall survival at 2 years (Non-small Cell Cancer Collaborative Group 1995). When this result is compared with CHART (Figure 4.3) it can be seen that the latter was almost twice as effective as the addition of chemotherapy to conventional radical treatment (Saunders et al. 1999).

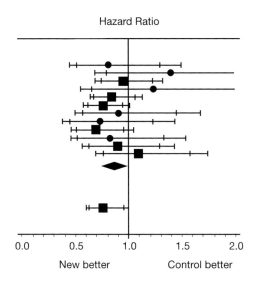

Figure 4.3 Results of the meta-analysis of randomised trials of cisplatin-based chemotherapy added to radiotherapy in non-small cell lung cancer compared with those of CHART.

This led the Department of Health, in its guidance for the treatment of non-small cell lung cancer, to recommend CHART as the treatment of choice for early inoperable disease (NHS Executive 1998). As implementation of the NHS guidelines was slow, a CHART implementation group was set up under the chairmanship of Dr Fergus Macbeth. The major problems identified as causing the slowness in uptake were:

- Cynicism among some consultant radiotherapists regarding the results of CHART trials and the advance it really represents. The maintenance of the benefit that has been shown in long-term follow-up is excellent support. However, it would be appropriate to ask the question whether the statistical significance translates into a real clinical advantage.

If we take the 2-year survival figures we find that, for CHART, it is 30% compared with 21% and at 5 years 12% compared with 7%. Even with CHART survival is poor and this must be faced; however, the 9% improvement at 2 years and the almost doubling of survival at 5 years represents the greatest advantage recorded in a trial in the management of locally advanced non-small cell lung cancer. Even though the treatment may be applicable to only a modest percentage of all newly presenting cases, perhaps 10%, when we consider the total of 40 000 new patients presenting annually in the UK, with over one million throughout the world, the increased survival possible with CHART could extend to a large number of people.

- It has been questioned whether CHART gives value for money. The survival curves have flattened after 3 years, suggesting that the advantage will continue over subsequent years. This has important consequences in determining life-years gained from the extra cost of providing CHART. Working with our colleague Søren Bentzen, we have calculated the cost per life gained to be £1300 at current values. By comparison with other health technologies, particularly those employed in cancer treatment, CHART is indeed a very economic proposal.

- There is a shortage of radiotherapy equipment in the UK which makes treating patients three times a day difficult, particularly because in most centres in the UK there are waiting lists for treatment. This has been exacerbated, particularly more recently, by a great shortage of radiographers.

The problem of treatment at the weekends was recognised early on and, indeed, many centres in Europe wished to take part in the randomised trial but could not treat on Saturdays and Sundays. CHART also presented a problem for dose escalation because it was not possible to do so without including a further weekend. Therefore, when the CHART trial began, those patients who were unsuitable for the trial were entered into a new pilot study – that of CHARTWEL (CHART **we**ekend-**le**ss) where we omitted weekend treatment and extended into a third week (see Figure 4.1). In this way we escalated the dose to 60 Gy. This regimen was tolerable, with no significant increase in acute or late morbidity and, although not strictly comparable because the cases were more advanced, the results were similar to those achieved in the CHART trial (Saunders et al. 1998).

Nevertheless, it is difficult to suggest that CHARTWEL should replace CHART in the treatment of non-small cell lung cancer, because there are no randomised controlled data to be evidence based. Currently, there are two trials comparing CHARTWEL to conventional radiotherapy: one in Europe and the other in the USA. The European trial, which has been pioneered by Professor Michael Baumann in Dresden, compares CHARTWEL to 60 Gy with conventional radiotherapy, in which a total dose of 66 Gy is given in 6.5 weeks. The dose of conventional radiotherapy has been raised because, since the inception of the CHART trials, conformal techniques of delivering radiotherapy have been introduced and these spare normal tissues; the 60 Gy, which was felt to be a suitable total dose for conventional treatment in 1990, is now not appropriate because it is felt that a higher dose should be achieved. In the USA a trial of CHARTWEL to 58.5 Gy is currently under way, comparing it to conventional radiotherapy 66 Gy in 6.5 weeks with neoadjuvant chemotherapy, using carboplatin and paclitaxel in both arms of the study (Herskovic et al. 1991). We are waiting for the studies to complete entry and to see the results.

It is, however, possible to make some theoretical predictions. In collaboration with Søren Bentzen, we have therefore modelled the likely effects of changing from CHART to CHARTWEL using human radiobiological data from the CHART studies and published radiobiological parameters for the normal tissues and tumours. There are three differences between CHART and CHARTWEL. First, the total dose has been raised from 54 Gy to 60 Gy, an 11% increase in dose which should be of benefit to tumour control. Second, the overall treatment time has been increased from 12 days to 18 days: this may be a slight disadvantage in terms of local tumour control if repopulation is taking place during that time. The third difference is that the weekends are omitted, which may lead to a reduction in late morbidity. In the modelling exercise, we have taken into account these three factors to try to predict the effect of CHARTWEL compared with CHART on the outcome in non-small cell lung cancer (Bentzen et al. 2002).

One of the most important factors will be the time of onset of repopulation and in particular if it begins before CHARTWEL is concluded. The data from Withers et al. (1988), but contested by Bentzen and Thames (1991), suggest that repopulation does not take place until the end of the third or beginning of the fourth week, and thus in the calculations that we have carried out we have looked at two scenarios: repopulation, first, beginning from the first day of treatment and, second, not commencing until after the first 3 weeks. It was possible for Søren Bentzen to calculate that CHARTWEL to 60 Gy was likely to improve tumour control in both scenarios, although there is uncertainty as to the degree of benefit. It could be predicted that tumour control at 3 years could increase by some 7–14 percentage points above the results of CHART, i.e. from 19% to between 26 and 33%, without significantly raising the level of acute or late morbidity (Bentzen et al. 2002).

In none of the modelling exercises was there any suggestion that CHARTWEL would be inferior to CHART. Therefore, in changing from CHART to CHARTWEL there may be a real increase in therapeutic benefit.

Conclusion

Radiobiological data, not only determined in non-small cell lung cancer but in other solid tumours, give good evidence that repopulation is an important cause of failure of radical radiotherapy. Accelerated schedules of radiotherapy have been extensively investigated at many sites and CHART has been the most successful in non-small cell lung cancer. It would seem reasonable, therefore, that centres look towards accelerated radiotherapy. Mathematical modelling would suggest that CHARTWEL is as good as CHART in improving the results of radiotherapy in non-small cell lung cancer.

In addition to the benefit gained by CHART we can take advantage of that suggested by the addition of cytotoxic chemotherapy. As CHART is given over short periods of time, it presents advantages over conventional radiotherapy when the combination of approaches is being tested. Initially, in pilot studies of chemotherapy combined with CHARTWEL, we gave neoadjuvant chemotherapy but are now moving forward to concomitant chemotherapy.

It will be important for the future that centres join together so that a combination of accelerated regimens, probably CHARTWEL, with chemotherapy can be tested in studies that accumulate adequate numbers of cases in a short period of time. The margins of advantage recently gained have been modest, but nevertheless they encourage us that, with further innovation, we can make more improvements and bring benefit to that previously undertreated group of patients – those with locally advanced non-small cell carcinoma.

Acknowledgements

I would like to acknowledge the assistance of Neeta Verma and Margaret Masters in producing this chapter.

References

Bennett MH, Wilson GD, Dische S, Saunders MI, Martindale CA, O'Halloran A (1992) Tumour proliferation assessed by combined histological and flow cytometric analysis: implications for therapy in squamous cell carcinoma in the head and neck. *British Journal of Cancer* **65**: 870–878.

Bentzen SM, Thames HD (1991) Clinical evidence for tumour clonogen regeneration: interpretations of the data. *Radiotherapy and Oncology* **22**: 161–166.

Bentzen S, Saunders MI, Dische S (2002) From CHART to CHARTWEL in non-small cell lung cancer. Clinical radiobiological modelling of the expected changes in outcome. *Clinical Oncology* in press.

Herskovic A. Orton C, Seyedsadr M et al. (1991) Initial experience with a practical hyperfractionated accelerated radiotherapy regimen. *International Journal of Radiation Oncology, Biology and Physics* **2**: 1275–1281.

NHS Executive (1998) *Guidance on Commissioning Cancer Services, Improving Outcomes in Lung Cancer. The Manual*. London: NHS Executive.

Non-small Cell Cancer Collaborative Group (1995) Chemotherapy in non-small cell lung cancer; a meta-analysis using updated data on individual patients from 52 randomised clinical trials. *British Medical Journal* **311**: 899–909.

Saunders M, Dische S (1990) Continuous, hyperfractionated, accelerated radiotherapy (CHART) in non-small cell carcinoma of the bronchus. *International Journal of Radiation Oncology, Biology and Physics* **19**: 1211–1215.

Saunders M, Dische S, Barrett A et al. (1996) Randomised multicentre trials of CHART vs conventional radiotherapy in head and neck and non-small cell lung cancer; an interim report. *British Journal of Cancer* **73**: 1455–1462.

Saunders M, Dische S, Barrett A et al. (1997) Continuous hyperfractionated accelerated radiotherapy (CHART) versus conventional radiotherapy in non-small cell lung cancer; a randomised multicentre trial. *The Lancet* **350**: 161–166.

Saunders MI, Rojas A, Lyn BE et al. (1998) Experience with dose escalation using CHARTWEL (Continuous Hyperfractionated Accelerated Radiotherapy Week-End Less) in non-small cell lung cancer. *British Journal of Cancer* **78**: 1323–1328.

Saunders M, Dische S, Barrett A et al. (1999) Continuous, hyperfractionated, accelerated radiotherapy (CHART) versus conventional radiotherapy in non-small cell lung cancer: Mature date from the randomised multicentre trial. *Radiotherapy and Oncology* **52**: 137–148.

Steele JD, Buell P (1971) Asymptomatic solitary pulmonary nodules: host survival, tumour site and growth rate. *Journal of Thoracic and Cardiovascular Surgery* **65**: 140–151.

Thames H, Withers H, Peters L, Fletcher G (1982) Changes in early and late radiation responses with altered dose fractionation: implications for dose–survival relationships. *International Journal of Radiation Oncology, Biology and Physics* **8**: 219–226.

Wilson GD, McNally NJ, Dische S et al. (1988) Measurement of cell kinetics in human tumours in vivo using bromodeoxyuridine incorporation and flow cytometry. *British Journal of Cancer* **58**: 423–431.

Withers HR, Thames HD, Peters LJ (1982) Differences in the fractionation response of acutely and late-responding tissues. In: Karcher KH, Kogelnik HD, Reinartz G (eds), *Progress in Radio-oncology II*. New York: Raven Press, pp. 287–296.

Withers HR, Taylor JMG, Maciejewski B (1988) The hazard of accelerated tumour clonogen repopulation during radiotherapy. *Acta Oncologica* **27**: 131–146.

Chapter 5

Scientific evidence and expert clinical opinion for medical intervention in early non-small cell lung cancer

Sarah Khan and Penella J Woll

The prognosis for patients with lung cancer remains poor, with overall 5-year survival rates varying from 12–15% in the USA to 5% in Scotland (Parkin et al. 1999; Gregor et al. 2001). Survival rates are strongly related to the stage of the disease at the time of diagnosis (Mountain 1997). Surgery is regarded as the best treatment option in patients with early stage non-small cell lung cancer (NSCLC); however, less than 20% of tumours are suitable for potentially curative resection (11% in Scotland – Gregor et al. 2001) and only about a third of these survive for 5 years. Radical radiotherapy is given with curative intent to patients who are medically inoperable or who refuse surgery, but in the UK this amounts to less than 5% of lung cancer patients (Gregor et al. 2001). Most patients will die with disseminated disease, so it is logical to use systemic therapy as early as possible to treat micrometastases.

There is good evidence that early tumours are more chemosensitive than advanced tumours, e.g. the response rate to MIC (mitomycin, ifosfamide, cisplatin) chemotherapy is 54% in regionally advanced NSCLC, but 32% in advanced disease (Cullen et al. 1999). In other tumour types, adjuvant and neoadjuvant chemotherapy have substantially improved the cure rates obtained by surgery or radiotherapy alone. The role of chemotherapy in early stage NSCLC has been questioned during 30 years of research. A meta-analysis including data from 9387 patients involved in 52 randomised clinical trials examined the effects of chemotherapy when combined with local treatment (surgery or radiotherapy). Most of the individual trials were too small for reliable detection of any significant differences between treatments, but even the meta-analysis proved inconclusive (NSCLC Collaborative Group 1995). Several larger studies have been published in the last 5 years and these are reviewed here.

This chapter will discuss the role of systemic chemotherapy in the management of early NSCLC by reviewing the role of multi-treatment modalities combining surgery, chemotherapy and radiotherapy, in the adjuvant and neoadjuvant setting. Literature searches were carried out on Medline, and published management guidelines have been referred to, including those of the American Society of Clinical Oncology, the UK Department of Health, The Royal College of Radiologists and the British Thoracic Society.

Combinations with surgery

All patients with early NSCLC (stage I and II) should be treated with complete surgical resection whenever possible (Korst and Ginsberg 2001). Up to 20% of patients present with tumours that may be suitable for potentially curative resection, but only 11% are currently operated on in the UK (Gregor et al. 2001). Although surgery achieves long-term survival in some patients, a significant proportion experience locoregional or distant recurrence (Pisters 2000). Five-year survival rates range from 60% for stage IA (T1N0M0) to 23% for stage IIB (T3N0M0 or T2N1M0) (Mountain 1997). The results of surgery in stage III patients are poor, especially for patients with N2 disease, of whom 85% will die from their disease in the 2 years after surgery. There is therefore scope to improve on the results of surgery, even in patients with stage I disease. Treatment failure is attributable to local recurrence in 30% of patients with the remainder re-presenting with metastatic disease.

Surgery and radiotherapy

Although most NSCLC patients die from disseminated disease, local recurrence is a common cause of first relapse. It is axiomatic to state that failure to achieve local tumour control will compromise survival and there are good data to show that improved local tumour control can improve overall survival (e.g. from the CHART study – Saunders et al. 1999). Two decades ago, many oncologists believed, from non-randomised trial data, that preoperative radiotherapy improved survival, albeit at the expense of loss of lung function and late cardiotoxicity. Eventually, three large phase III studies were conducted, none of which showed any advantage for preoperative radiotherapy compared with surgery alone (Einhorn 1998).

Similarly, postoperative radiotherapy was expected to be superior to surgery alone, until the Lung Cancer Study Group's randomised phase III trial of 210 patients with resectable stage IIA/IIIA disease demonstrated otherwise. The study showed a significant reduction in local recurrence rates to the ipsilateral lung and mediastinum in patients receiving postoperative radiotherapy, but no overall survival advantage. Overall recurrence rates were reduced by radiotherapy in patients with N2 disease ($p < 0.05$), although this subgroup had no evidence of improved survival (Lung Cancer Study Group 1987). The PORT (postoperative radiotherapy) Meta-Analysis Trialists Group (1998) carried out a meta-analysis of nine randomised control trials involving 2128 patients. All patients had completely resected tumours with disease stage no greater than IIIA. Radiotherapy doses ranged from 30 to 60 Gy given in 10–30 fractions and there was considerable variability in other aspects of the radiotherapy planning. There was clear evidence of a detrimental effect of PORT on survival. The 21% relative increase in death associate with PORT (hazard ratio 1.21; 95% confidence interval or 95%CI 1.08–1.34) was equivalent to an overall reduction in survival from 55% to 48% at 2 years ($p = 0.001$), which was most pronounced in stage I/II patients, and was attributable to excess early and late cardiopulmonary toxicity. There was also a lesser adverse effect on local, distant and overall recurrence-free survival. Overall, PORT cannot be recommended for stage I/II NSCLC.

Surgery and postoperative chemotherapy

The modest long-term survival rates obtained with surgery alone in early stage NSCLC prompted studies of adjuvant (postoperative) chemotherapy. There is accumulating evidence to suggest that NSCLC is a systemic disease from presentation, e.g. cytokeratin-positive micrometastases can be detected in the bone marrow in 54% of N0 patients (Pantel et al. 1996).

A number of studies using adjuvant chemotherapy in early stage NSCLC have given encouraging early results, e.g. Niiranen and colleagues (1992) randomised 110 patients with stage I NSCLC to treatment with chemotherapy (six cycles of cyclophosphamide, doxorubicin and cisplatin) or no additional treatment after radical surgery. Progression rates were lower in the chemotherapy arm (31% vs 48%, $p = 0.01$) and the survival rate at 10 years was higher in the chemotherapy arm (61% vs 48%, $p = 0.05$).

The NSCLC Collaborative Group Meta-Analysis (1995) included 4357 patients in 14 randomised trials of surgery versus surgery + chemotherapy. In trials using long-term alkylating agents, adjuvant chemotherapy was detrimental to survival (hazard ratio 1.15, 95%CI 1.04–1.27, $p = 0.005$), leading to a 4% survival reduction at 2 years. In contrast, cisplatin-containing adjuvant chemotherapy improved survival (hazard ratio 0.87, 95%CI 0.74–1.02, $p = 0.08$), leading to a 3% survival benefit at 2 years and an absolute benefit of 5% at 5 years.

However, a Japanese study that has recently been reported in abstract suggests that postoperative chemotherapy adds no advantage in patients who have had a pathological complete resection (Ichinose et al. 2001); 119 patients with stage IIIA, N2 NSCLC were radically resected, and then randomised to receive three cycles of cisplatin/vindesine chemotherapy or no additional treatment. The median survival (35 months) and 3-year survival rate (49%) were identical in the two groups.

Based on this evidence, postoperative chemotherapy cannot be routinely recommended and should be given only in a clinical trial, such as the UK Big Lung Trial.

Surgery and preoperative chemotherapy

Postoperative chemotherapy is attractive because it does not delay the definitive treatment or increase the morbidity of surgery. There is, however, often a significant delay in starting adjuvant chemotherapy to allow for healing after thoracotomy, which may abrogate the benefits of treating micrometastases early. Preoperative (neoadjuvant) chemotherapy has therefore been proposed in order to expose micrometastases to drugs as early as possible, while the vasculature is still intact, and to shrink tumours before surgery (Klastersky et al. 1991; Pastorino 1996). Surgeons are understandably sceptical about the risks of delaying surgery and increasing perioperative morbidity and mortality. Some tumours will progress despite early chemotherapy and may become irresectable, but such aggressive tumours were unlikely to be cured by surgery alone. Another difficulty is in knowing how much to resect in cases where major tumour shrinkage has been achieved with chemotherapy.

Numerous phase II studies of preoperative chemotherapy have been published, most in stage III tumours. Preoperative chemotherapy may increase resection rates in stage IIIA disease, but there are no well-defined criteria for resectability, nor is there a consensus about the best schedule for preoperative chemotherapy. Four randomised studies comparing cisplatin-based chemotherapy plus surgery versus surgery alone in stage IIIA disease have been published, all showing a survival advantage to preoperative chemotherapy (Table 5.1).

Two influential studies were first published in 1994 (Rosell et al. 1994; Roth et al. 1994). Both were randomised studies of preoperative chemotherapy in patients with stage IIIA NSCLC. In both, recruitment was closed prematurely after 60 patients had been entered, because of a large survival difference between the two arms. This has reduced their statistical power and made exploratory subgroup analysis impossible. Inevitably, longer follow-up has narrowed the gap between the treatment arms. In the Spanish study (Rosell et al. 1994, 1999), 60 patients were randomised to surgery alone or to receive three cycles of MIC chemotherapy (cisplatin 50 mg/m^2) followed by surgery. In addition, all patients received thoracic radiation, as 50 Gy in 25 fractions over 5 weeks. The median survival was initially reported to be 26 months in the chemotherapy group and 8 months in the control group ($p < 0.001$), with a median disease-free survival of 20 versus 5 months. With longer follow-up, however, the median survival was 22 months in the chemotherapy group and 10 months in the control group ($p < 0.001$), with 17% and 0% alive at 5 years (Rosell et al. 1999). The trial has been criticised for patient heterogeneity and the poor outcome in the surgery-alone group. A further study by Rosell conducted in stage IIIA N2 disease compared treatment with chemotherapy containing cisplatin 50 and 100 mg/m^2. This achieved median survivals of 11 months and 12 months respectively (Rosell et al. 1996).

In the Texan study (Roth et al. 1994, 1998), 60 patients with stage IIIA NSCLC were randomised to surgery alone or to receive three cycles of CEP (cyclophosphamide, etoposide, cisplatin) chemotherapy (cisplatin 100 mg/m^2) followed by surgery. The median survival was initially reported to be 64 months in the chemotherapy group and 11 months in the control group ($p < 0.008$), with a 3-year survival rate of 56% versus 15%. With longer follow-up, however, the median survival was 21 months in the chemotherapy group and 14 months in the control group ($p < 0.05$), with 36% and 15% alive at 5 years (Roth et al. 1998). The preliminary results of these

Table 5.1 Randomised studies of preoperative chemotherapy for NSCLC

Authors	Patient number	Chemotherapy regimen	Stage	Response rate (%)	pCR rate (%)	Resection rate (S/C + S)	Operative mortality (S/C + S)	Median survival (months) (S/C + S)
Pass et al. (1992)	27	EP	IIIA, N2	61	7.6	86/85	0	15.6/28.7 p = 0.09
Rosell et al. (1994, 1999)	60	MIP	IIIA	53	3.3	90/85	6.6/6.6	10/22 p = 0.05
Roth et al. (1994, 1998)	60	CEP	IIIA	35	3.6	66/61	6/3	14/21 p = 0.05
Depierre et al. (1999)	375	MIP	IB, II, IIIA	53	11	86/92	4.5/7.8	26/37 p = 0.009

pCR, pathological complete response; S, surgery; C + S, chemotherapy and surgery; mo, months; C, cyclophosphamide; E, etoposide; P, cisplatin; M, mitomycin; I, ifosfamide.

two studies were published in prominent journals and aroused tremendous interest in the use of preoperative chemotherapy for NSCLC, leading to the initiation of several studies worldwide.

From 1991 to 1997, The French Co-operative Oncology Group conducted a randomised study in 373 stage I/II/III resectable NSCLC patients, comparing preoperative chemotherapy and surgery to surgery alone. Preliminary results were reported at the American Society of Clinical Oncology (ASCO – Depierre et al. 1999). Two cycles of MIP chemotherapy were given preoperatively at 3-week intervals, with a further two cycles postoperatively. In both arms, postoperative radiotherapy was given to patients with pT3 or N2 disease. Higher perioperative toxicity was noted in patients who had received chemotherapy. The median survival was 37 months in the preoperative chemotherapy arm and 26 months in the control arm; 2- and 3-year survival rates were 59% and 52% versus 52% and 41% in the control arm.

Thus preliminary evidence suggests that preoperative chemotherapy can improve the results of surgery, but it is not yet clear whether the benefits apply equally to stage I and stage IIIA patients. Nor has the best chemotherapy regimen been defined yet. Considerable concerns remain about the risk of worse perioperative morbidity and mortality after chemotherapy (Siegenthaler et al. 2001). This will be better defined when ongoing studies are reported, e.g. the Spanish Lung Cancer Group (SLCG) is currently conducting a trial comparing three treatment arms in patients with stage Ia, IIA and IIB NSCLC: preoperative chemotherapy followed by surgery, surgery alone and surgery plus postoperative chemotherapy. Preoperative chemotherapy is not recommended for routine use, but all operable patients should be offered the opportunity of discussing ongoing clinical trials, such as the UK Medical Research Council LU22 study.

Surgery, radiotherapy and chemotherapy

The NSCLC Collaborative Group Meta-Analysis (1995) included 807 patients in 7 randomised trials of surgery + radiotherapy versus surgery + radiotherapy + chemotherapy. Six of the studies used cisplatin-containing regimens. There was considerable variability in doses and schedules for both radiotherapy and chemotherapy, making interpretation difficult. Although the hazard ratios were marginally in favour of chemotherapy, the confidence intervals were wide (hazard ratio 0.94, 95%CI 0.79–1.11, for cisplatin-based chemotherapy).

To elucidate the role of chemotherapy in resectable NSCLC, the Eastern Co-operative Group (ECOG) undertook a large randomised study of postoperative radiotherapy versus postoperative radiotherapy and chemotherapy (Keller et al. 2000); 488 patients with stage II–IIIA NSCLC were randomised to 50.4 Gy in 28 fractions with or without etoposide/cisplatin 60 mg/m^2 for four cycles. The overall median survival was 38 months in both arms, suggesting no advantage for the addition of chemoradiation in the management of resectable (stage II/IIIA) NSCLC.

A German study of postoperative chemoradiotherapy has been reported in abstract (Wolf et al. 2001). Patients with completely resected N2 NSCLC were randomised to receive either radiotherapy alone (50 Gy in 5 weeks) or three cycles of cisplatin/ ifosfamide chemotherapy followed by the same radiotherapy. The study was closed after 150 of the planned 300 patients had been randomised, because of slow accrual and identical median survival (34 months) and 3-year survival rates (46%) in the two groups.

The role of postoperative chemoradiotherapy for NSCLC remains highly controversial. It cannot be routinely recommended.

Combinations with radiotherapy

Among patients with stage I–II NSCLC, there are a number who, although technically resectable, either refuse surgery or are considered inoperable as a result of insufficient respiratory reserve, cardiovascular disease or general frailty. Such patients are considered medically inoperable and, although there is no evidence from randomised trials supporting the use of radical radiotherapy in stage I/II NSCLC, most clinical oncologists believe that these patients should receive radical (as opposed to palliative) radiotherapy (Royal College of Radiologists' Clinical Information Network 1999). Some stage IIIA patients who are irresectable can also be considered for radical radiotherapy.

The outcome of patients treated with radical radiotherapy lies between that of patients treated with surgery and those who are untreated. It is also influenced by the presence of co-morbidities, including chronic obstructive pulmonary disease (COPD) and coronary artery disease, which most commonly render patients inoperable (Rowell and Williams 2001). Comparisons are difficult, however, because of stage definition: the 5-year survival rate in surgically staged patients is 67% for T1N0 (stage IA) and 57% for T2N0 (stage IB) tumours, but 61% and 38% respectively in clinically staged tumours (Mountain 1997). In those patients with involved hilar nodes (stage IIA), 5-year survival rates were 55% and 39% for T1N1 and T2N1, respectively, in the pathologically staged group, and 34% and 24% in the clinically staged group.

Radical radiotherapy for NSCLC usually consists of approximately 60 Gy delivered to the midplane of the volume of known tumour, using conventional fractionation. A boost to the primary tumour is frequently used to further enhance local control. Continuous hyperfractionated accelerated radiotherapy (CHART) was shown to give better overall survival than conventional radical radiotherapy in a randomised trial including 563 patients with stage I–IIIB NSCLC (Saunders et al. 1999) and has been recommended in the UK by the Department of Health and The Royal College of Radiologists' guidelines. In this study, the 3-year survival rate for radical radiotherapy using CHART was 20%.

Chemotherapy and radiotherapy

Radical radiotherapy remains the mainstay of treatment for inoperable NSCLC, but its curative potential is low. Therefore, a number of studies have been performed to determine whether the use of chemoradiotherapy improves survival compared with radiotherapy alone.

Many early studies comparing radiation alone with radiation and chemotherapy were negative or inconclusive. The NSCLC Collaborative Group Meta-analysis (1995) included 3033 patients in 22 trials comparing radical radiotherapy with radical radiotherapy plus chemotherapy. It showed a significant overall benefit from chemotherapy (hazard ratio 0.90, $p = 0.006$), corresponding to an absolute survival benefit of 3% at 2 years. In these studies, chemotherapy with alkylating agents was not detrimental but, once again, the strongest evidence of benefit was seen in the 1780 patients enrolled in 11 trials using cisplatin-based chemotherapy (hazard ratio 0.87, 95%CI 0.79–0.96 ($p = 0.005$)), corresponding to an absolute survival benefit of 4% at 2 years. This meta-analysis included both sequential and concurrent chemoradiation studies.

Sequential chemotherapy and radiotherapy

A number of phase III trials have compared sequential chemoradiotherapy with radiotherapy alone (Table 5.2). Several earlier studies did not show a significant advantage for combined modality treatment, but three large phase III trials (two from the USA and one from France) showed statistically significant results in favour of combined treatment. The CALGB group (Cancer and Leukaemia Group B) randomly assigned 155 patients with locally advanced NSCLC (stage III), to either radiotherapy alone (60 Gy over 6 weeks) or the same radiotherapy preceded by two cycles of cisplatin and vinblastine. The first report of the study showed that 23% of patients receiving combined modality treatment were still alive after 3 years compared with 11% of those receiving radiotherapy alone (Dillman et al. 1990). The survival benefit was maintained after 7 years of follow-up (Dillman et al. 1996). Similar results were found in the French study (Le Chevalier et al. 1991, 1992). The largest study was that of the Radiotherapy Oncology Group (RTOG) in which 490 patients were randomised to standard or hyperfractionated radiation, or sequential chemoradiotherapy (Sause et al. 1995, 2000). Both the median survival and the 2-year survival were significantly higher in the chemoradiotherapy than the conventional radiotherapy arm. A British study was less clear-cut in its results: 446 patients with locally advanced disease were randomly assigned radiotherapy (at least 40 Gy in 15 fractions) or the same radiotherapy preceded by four cycles of MIC chemotherapy. The difference in median survival of 2 months in favour of the chemotherapy group was not statistically significant (Cullen et al. 1999). This study has been criticised for suboptimal radiation treatment, which may have compromised the results.

Table 5.2 Phase III studies of sequential chemotherapy and radiation versus radiation alone in NSCLC

Authors	Patient number	Therapy	Median survival (months)	2-year survival rate (%)	p
Mattson et al. (1988)	238	55 Gy ± Cyclophosphamide, doxorubicin, cisplatin	10 11	17 19	NS
Morton et al. (1991)	114	60 Gy ± Methotrexate, doxorubicin, cyclophosphamide, etoposide	10 10	16 21	NS
Le Chevalier et al. (1991, 1992)	353	65 Gy in 26 fractions ± Cisplatin, vinblastine, etoposide, cyclophosphamide 10	10 12	14 21	<0.05
Dillman et al. (1990, 1996)	155	60 Gy in 30 fractions ± Cisplatin, vinblastine	9.7 13.8	13 26	0.012
Sause et al. (1995, 2000)	458	60 Gy in 30 fractions or 69.6 Gy HFX as 1.2 Gy twice daily ± Cisplatin, vinblastine	11.4 12 13.2	21 24 32	0.04
Brodin et al. (1996)	302	56 Gy, 2 Gy/day ± Cisplatin, etoposide	11 11	17 21	NS
Cullen et al. (1999)	446	At least 40 Gy in 15 fractions ± Cisplatin, mitomycin, ifosfamide	9.7 11.7	16 20	NS

RT, radiotherapy; CT, chemotherapy; HFX, hyperfractionated; NS, not statistically significant.

The European Lung Cancer Working Party study compared radiotherapy with maintenance chemotherapy in patients responding to primary chemotherapy; 115 NSCLC patients who responded to primary chemotherapy were randomly assigned further chemotherapy or chest irradiation (60 Gy over 6 weeks). Despite better control in the radiotherapy group, there was no significant difference in survival (Sculier et al. 1999). Patients with chemoresponsive N2 disease should be considered for randomisation in a study such as the European Organisation for the Research and Treatment of Cancer (EORTC) study 08941, which compares consolidation radiotherapy with surgery.

Concurrent chemotherapy and radiotherapy

It has been known for many years that some cytotoxic agents are radiosensitising, and concurrent chemoradiotherapy has been used in a number of tumour types to take advantage of this effect (e.g. Rose et al. 1999). Typically, chemotherapy drugs are given in low doses daily or weekly throughout the course of radiotherapy, with the dual intention of optimising disease control and treating micrometastases early. Unfortunately, the concurrent use of chemotherapy and radiotherapy also leads to increased toxicity in normal tissues, which may compromise the delivery of full-dose radiotherapy. Table 5.3 shows the published phase III studies of concomitant chemoradiation versus radiation alone. Most studies do not show a statistically significant difference in survival between patients treated with concomitant chemoradiation versus radiation alone; however, four regimens did result in a significant difference in 2-year survival.

Sequential and concurrent chemoradiotherapy have been compared in two major cooperative group, randomised, phase III trials, which have demonstrated superior survival in patients with locally advanced, unresectable NSCLC receiving concurrent chemoradiotherapy (Furuse et al. 1999; Curran et al. 2000). In the first, from Japan, 320 patients with stage III NSCLC were randomised to receive two cycles of MVC (mitomycin, vindesine, cisplatin) chemotherapy followed by chest irradiation (56 Gy in 28 fractions), or the same chemotherapy given together with radiotherapy (Furuse et al. 1999). The study showed a significant survival advantage in the concomitant arm (16.5 months vs 13.3 months, $p = 0.04$) but at the expense of more myelosuppression (Furuse et al. 1999). These results were similar to the RTOG study involving 611 patients, who were randomised to three arms, sequential chemotherapy with vinblastine/cisplatin followed by standard daily fraction radiotherapy (Seq), concurrent chemoradiotherapy with vinblastine/cisplatin (Con-QD) or hyperfractionated radiotherapy and concurrent cisplatin/etoposide (Con-BID). Relative median survival for the Seq, Con-QD and Con-BID were 14.5, 17 and 15.6 months, respectively. At the time of analysis, there was a statistically significant advantage for Con-QD ($p = 0.038$). Unsurprisingly, toxicities were worse in the concurrent arms (Curran et al. 2000).

Table 5.3 Phase III studies of concomitant chemoradiation versus radiation alone in NSCLC

Authors	Patient number	Therapy	Median survival (months)	2-year survival rate (%)	p
Schaake-Koning et al. (1992)	308	RT	12	13	
		RT + daily cisplatin	14	26	0.009
		RT + weekly cisplatin	12	19	NS
Trovo et al. (1992)	169	RT	10	13	
		RT + daily cisplatin	10	13	NS
Ball et al. (1999)	204	RT	14	26	
		HFX RT	14	28	NS
		RT + carboplatin	17	29	
		HFX RT + carboplatin	15	20	
Clamon et al. (1999)	250	RT	13	26	
		RT + carboplatin	13	29	NS
Blanke et al. (1995)	215	RT	10	13	
		RT + cisplatin q 3 wks	11	18	NS
Trovo et al. (1990)	111	RT	12	17	
		RT + MTX/dox/cyclo	10	19	0.003
Jeremic et al. (1995)	169	HFX RT	8	25	
		HFX RT + carboplatin/etop (low dose)	18	35	0.003
Jeremic et al. (1993)	131	HFX RT + carboplatin/etop (high dose)	13	27	NS
		HFX RT	14	26	0.021
		HFX RT + carboplatin/etop (daily)	22	43	

RT, radiotherapy; CT, chemotherapy; HFX, hyperfractionated; MTX, methotrexate; cyclo, cyclophosphamide; dox, doxorubicin; etop, etoposide.

The choice of chemotherapy regimen to be used in combination with radiotherapy is not clear. Most of the existing data are for cisplatin-containing regimens and there are few data on the newer agents such as the taxanes, vinorelbine, gemcitabine or topoisomerase inhibitors. Preliminary data are available from the South-West Oncology Group (SWOG) study 9504 (Gaspar et al. 2001); 83 patients with stage IIIB NSCLC were treated with concurrent radiotherapy (61 Gy), etoposide (50 mg/m^2 days 1–5, 29–33) and cisplatin (50 mg/m^2 days 1, 8, 29, 36) followed by 'consolidation' docetaxel (75–100 mg/m^2 every 21 days) for three cycles. Preliminary data were reported last year, when the projected mean survival was 22 months. The median follow-up is now 28 months, with an improvement in median survival of 27 months. A 3-year survival rate of 40% was reported with the docetaxel-containing regimen compared with 17% in the historical controls using cisplatin and etoposide.

Although the survival benefits are modest, combined modality approaches using chemotherapy and radiotherapy are standard in many centres in selected patients and were recommended by the ASCO Guidelines (1997). Despite additional morbidity, concomitant treatment seems to provide better locoregional tumour control and overall survival. There are no randomised studies testing the combination of chemotherapy with CHART. If they can be successfully combined, this approach could offer greater survival gains than combining chemotherapy with conventional radiotherapy.

Biological agents in early NSCLC

Many biological agents have been studied in the treatment of early stage NSCLC, including BCG (Bacille Calmette–Guérin), levamisole, *Corynebacterium parvum*, interferons, tumour necrosis factor (TNF) and specific lymphokine-activated cell therapy; however, results to date have been disappointing (Table 5.4) (Shepherd 1997). Current research is focusing on the development of signal transduction inhibitors, cell cycle regulatory compounds, immunomodulators and anti-angiogenesis agents.

The EGFR (epidermal growth factor receptor) pathway contributes to the aggressiveness of many tumour types, and is over-expressed in 40–80% of cases of NSCLC. A number of drugs have been developed that target the EGF receptor, including blocking antibodies (e.g. C225) and EGFR tyrosine kinase inhibitors (e.g. iressa, ZD1839) which have shown interesting results in early clinical studies (Hong et al. 2001; Miller et al. 2001; Perez-Soler et al. 2001). Synergy exists between these compounds and standard chemotherapeutic agents, and may give an enhanced anti-tumour effect. They are currently being tested as adjuncts to chemotherapy in patients with advanced NSCLC.

Similarly, the matrix metalloproteases, such as Marimastat and Prinomastat, and immunotherapies such as *Mycobacterium vaccae* (SRL) have shown interesting

Table 5.4 Randomised studies of biological agents used adjuvantly in NSCLC

Author	Patient number	Therapy	Outcome
Gail (1994)	473	Surgery ± intrapleural BCG	No significant difference
Holmes (1994)	141	Surgery ± intrapleural BCG	Better disease-free survival with CAP
Anthony et al. (1979)	318	Surgery + CAP or BCG/levamisole	Excess deaths in levamisole group
Amery (1978)	211	Surgery ± levamisole	No significant difference
Ludwig Lung Cancer Study Group (1985)	475	Intrapleural and intravenous *Corynebacterium parvum*	Adverse effect with biological therapy
Lee et al. (1994)	93	Surgery ± intrapleural *Streptococcus pyogenes*	No significant difference
Whyte et al. (1992)	63	Surgery/RT ± transfer factor	Non-significant survival benefit
Hollinshead et al. (1987)	234	Surgery ± adjuvant ± vaccine	Improved survival with vaccine
Takita et al. (1991)	85	Surgery ± specific immunotherapy	Improved survival with immunotherapy

BCG, Bacillus Calmette–Guérin; CAP, cyclophosphamide, doxorubicin, cisplatin; RT, radiotherapy.

activity in uncontrolled studies, and are now being tested in combination with chemotherapy in patients with advanced NSCLC.

The future

Newer cytotoxic drugs

Results to date suggest that the addition of systemic therapies to conventional surgery and radiotherapy may improve survival rates. Trials currently in progress should help define the best ways of combining these treatment modalities. All of the reliable data so far use cisplatin-containing regimens. Newer agents, including docetaxel, paclitaxel, gemcitabine, vinorelbine and the topoisomerase inhibitors, have good activity in advanced NSCLC and the first three of these have recently been recommended by the National Institute for Clinical Excellence (NICE) for use in the UK in this setting (NICE 2001). There are insufficient data to recommend their use in early disease, although their use is being tested in several ongoing studies.

Docetaxel has been incorporated into several neoadjuvant regimens (Rosell 1999). One randomised study has been reported in abstract that is of particular interest in using a non-platinum regimen (Mattson et al. 2000): 274 patients with radically treatable stage IIIA–B NSCLC were randomised to receive local treatment alone (surgery or radiotherapy, decided before study entry) or prior therapy using three cycles of single-agent docetaxel 100 mg/m^2. As expected, higher response rates were obtained in earlier stage disease (37% for IIB–IIIA T3, 35% for IIIA N2 and 21% for IIIB). The preliminary results demonstrate a survival advantage for neoadjuvant docetaxel (median survival 15.6 vs 13.7 months, 1 year survival rate 60% vs 56%) which is evident for each stage group, but mature data and toxicity data are not yet available.

Newer biological approaches

Lung cancer arises from a multistep process resulting in the accumulation of genetic alterations in cells (Hirsch et al. 2001). Both genetic (e.g. allelic losses at chromosomes 3p, 9p, 8p, 17p and *MYC*, *RAS* and *P53* mutations) and epigenetic alterations (e.g. inactivating methylation of tumour-suppressor genes) are thought to occur. It is likely that, in the future, molecular information will be incorporated into the staging formulation at the time of diagnosis. The use of molecular markers as a means of detecting minimal residual disease after apparent complete response is also likely to influence patient management. The genotypical abnormalities in an individual tumour (such as *P53*, EGFR or *CYP3A* status) may predict not only overall prognosis, but also the likelihood of response to particular cytotoxics or biological agents. An ongoing trial (Genotypic International Lung Trial) is testing potential molecular predictive factors in order to optimise currently available therapy in individual patients and patient subsets.

As noted above, the biology of lung cancer is a rapidly developing field, and new discoveries are revealing new targets for novel therapeutic approaches. Those currently under investigation include signal transduction inhibitors, cell cycle regulatory compounds, immunomodulators and anti-angiogenesis agents. The optimal use for many of these agents will be in combination with chemotherapy or radiotherapy, or after cytoreduction from surgery or combined modality treatment.

Conclusion

Although the survival rates of patients who present with early stage NSCLC remain disappointingly low, much effort has been directed to improving this. There is no doubt that surgery offers the best hope of cure in patients with early stage disease. Recurrence rates, however, are high. Even among the élite with stage IA disease, a third of patients relapse and die of their disease within 5 years. Intrathoracic relapses occur in a third whereas distant relapses occur in two-thirds of these patients – hence the enthusiasm for testing the use of systemic therapy in early stage NSCLC. For patients with stage I or II NSCLC, there is preliminary evidence of survival benefits from preoperative or postoperative chemotherapy, but further data are needed to evaluate whether these benefits are clinically significant or outweighed by increased toxicity.

The optimal management of patients with stage III NSCLC remains controversial. Potential roles exist for surgery, radiotherapy and chemotherapy, but there is no standard of treatment performed. Some of the uncertainty arises from the difficulty of establishing the nodal stage, particularly in centres where mediastinoscopy and/or positron emission tomography are not routinely available. Postoperative adjuvant chemotherapy has not shown any clear impact on survival and further research is needed in this area. Neoadjuvant chemotherapy is being used in stage IIIA NSCLC in the hope of downsizing tumours to make them operable, but this will not necessarily improve survival. The use of concurrent chemoradiation has been shown in several studies to be beneficial when compared with radiation alone, or sequential chemoradiotherapy in patients with unresectable tumours, and is the treatment of choice in many centres across the world, particularly the USA (ASCO 1997).

Present and future studies will focus on the role of both new cytotoxics and new biological agents. At present, the best advice to clinicians and patients is that cancer patients treated in clinical trials have better outcomes than those off-study, so all patients with early NSCLC should be offered entry into clinical trials in order to evaluate the most appropriate treatment modality.

References

American Society of Clinical Oncology (1997) Clinical practice guidelines for the treatment of unresectable non-small-cell lung cancer. *Journal of Clinical Oncology* **15**: 2996–3018.

Amery WK (1978) Final results of a multicenter placebo-controlled levamisole study of resectable lung cancer. *Cancer Treatment Report* **62**: 1671–1683.

Anthony HM, Mearns AJ, Mason MK et al. (1979) Levamisole in surgery of bronchogenic carcinoma patients: increased deaths from cardiorespiratory failure. *Thorax* **34**: 4–12.

Ball D, Bishop J, Smith J et al. (1999) A randomised phase III study of accelerated or standard fraction radiotherapy with or without concurrent carboplatin in inoperable non-small cell lung cancer: final report of an Australian multi-centre trial. *Radiotherapeutic Oncology* **52**: 129–136.

Blanke C, Ansari R, Montravadi R et al. (1995) A phase III trial of thoracic irradiation with and without concomitant cisplatin for locally advanced unresectable non-small cell lung cancer: A Hoosier Group Oncology Group Study. *Journal of Clinical Oncology* **13**: 1425–1429.

Brodin O, Nou E, Mercke C et al. (1996) Comparison of induction chemotherapy before radiotherapy with radiotherapy only in patients with locally advanced squamous cell carcinoma of the lung. *European Journal of Cancer* **32A**: 1893–1890.

Clamon G, Herndon J, Cooper R et al. (1999) Radiosensitisation with carboplatin for patients with unresectable stage III NSCLC: a phase III trial of the Cancer and Leukemia Group B and the Eastern Cooperative Oncology Group. *Journal of Clinical Oncology* **17**: 4–11.

Cullen MH, Billingham LJ, Quoix E et al. (1999) Mitomycin, ifosfamide and cisplatin in unresectable non-small-cell lung cancer: effects on survival and quality of life. *Journal of Clinical Oncology* **17**: 3188–3194.

Curran WJ, Scott C, Langer C et al. (2000) RTOG 9410: Concurrent versus asynchronous chemoradiotherapy in NSCLC. *Proceedings of the American Society of Clinical Oncology* **19**: 1484–1489.

Department of Health (1997) *Improving Outcomes in Lung Cancer*. London: DoH.

Depierre A, Milleron B, Moro D et al. (1999) Phase III trial of neoadjuvant chemotherapy in resectable stage I,II and III NSCLC: the French experience. *Proceedings of the American Society of Clinical Oncology* **18**: 465a (abstract 1792).

Dillman RO, Seagren SL, Herndon J et al. (1990) A randomised trial of induction chemotherapy plus high dose radiotherapy vs. radiotherapy alone in stage III non-small-cell lung cancer. *New England Journal of Medicine* **329**: 940–945.

Dillman RO, Herndon J, Seagren SL et al. (1996) Improved survival in stage III NSCLC: seven year follow up of CALGB 8433 trial. *Journal of the National Cancer Institute* **88**: 1210–1214.

Einhorn LH (1988) Neoadjuvant therapy of stage III NSCLC. *Annals of Thoracic Surgery* **46**: 362–365.

Furuse K, Fukuoka M, Kawahara M et al. (1999) Phase III study of concurrent versus sequential thoracic radiotherapy in combination with mitomycin, vindesine and cisplatin in unresectable stage III NSCLC: five year median follow-up results. *Journal of Clinical Oncology* **17**: 2692–2699.

Gai MH (1994) A placebo-controlled randomised double-blind study of adjuvant intrapleural BCG in patients with resected T1N0, T1N1 or T2N0 squamous cell carcinoma, adenocarcinoma, or large cell carcinoma of the lung. LCSG Protocol-771. *Chest* **106**(6): S287–S292 suppl.

Gaspar L, Gandara D, Chansky K et al. (2001) Consolidation docetaxel following concurrent chemoradiotherapy in pathologic stage IIIB non-small cell lung cancer (SWOG 9504): patterns of failure and updated survival. *Proceedings of the American Society of Clinical Oncology* **20**: abstract 1255.

Gregor A, Thomson CS, Brewster DH et al. (2001) Management and survival of patients with lung cancer in Scotland diagnosed in 1995: results of a national population based study. *Thorax* **56**: 212–217.

Hirsch FR, Franklin WA, Gazdar AF, Bunn PA (2001) Early detection of lung cancer; clinical perspectives of recent advances in biology and radiology. *Clinical Cancer Research* **7**: 5–22.

Hollinshead A, Stewart THM, Takita H, Dalbow M, Concannon J (1987) Adjuvant specific active lung cancer immunotherapy trials. *Cancer* **60**: 1249.

Holmes EC (1994) Surgical adjuvant therapy for stage-II and stage-III adenocarcinoma and large cell undifferentiated carcinoma. *Chest* **106**(6): S293–S296 suppl.

Hong WK, Arquette M, Nabell L et al. (2001) Efficacy and safety of anti-epidermal growth factor antibody (EGFR) IMC-C225, in combination with cisplatin in patients with recurrent squamous cell carcinoma of head and neck refractory to cisplatin containing chemotherapy. *Proceedings of the American Society of Clinical Oncology* **20**: 224a (abstract 895).

Ichinose Y, Tada H, Koike T et al. (2001) A randomised phase III trial of post operative adjuvant chemotherapy in patients with completely resected stage IIIA-N2 NSCLC; Japan Clinical Oncology Group (JCOG 9304) Trial. *Proceedings of the American Society of Clinical Oncology* **20**: abstract 1241.

Jeremic B, Jevremovic S, Mijatovic L et al. (1993) Hyperfractionated radiation therapy with and without concurrent chemotherapy for advanced NSCLC. *Cancer* **71**: 3732–3736.

Jeremic B, Shibamoto Y, Acimovic L et al. (1995) Randomised trial of hyperfractionated radiation therapy with or without concurrent chemotherapy for stage III NSCLC. *Journal of Clinical Oncology* **13**: 452–458.

Jeremic B, Shibamoto Y, Acimovic L et al. (1996) Hyperfractionated radiation therapy with or without concurrent low-dose daily carboplatin/etoposide for stage III NSCLC: a randomised study. *Journal of Clinical Oncology* **14**: 1065–1070.

Johnson H, Einhorn LH, Bartolucci A et al. (1990) Thoracic radiotherapy does not prolong survival in patients with locally advanced unresectable no-small cell lung cancer. *Annals of Internal Medicine* **113**: 33–38.

Keller SM, Adak S, Wagner H et al. (2000) A randomised trial of postoperative adjuvant therapy in patients with completely resected stage II or IIIA non-small cell lung cancer. *New England Journal of Medicine* **343**: 1217–1222.

Klastersky J, Burkers R, Choi N et al. (1991) Induction therapy for NSCLC. A consensus report. *Lung Cancer* **7**: 15–17.

Korst RJ, Ginsberg RJ (2001) Appropriate management of resectable NSCLC. *World Journal of Surgery* **25**: 184–188.

Le Chevalier T, Arriagada R, Quoix E et al. (1991) Radiotherapy alone versus combined chemotherapy and radiotherapy in nonresectable non-small cell lung cancer: first analysis of a randomised trial in 353 patients. *Journal of the National Cancer Institute* **83**: 17–23.

Le Chevalier T, Arriagada R, Tarayre M et al. (1992) Significant effect of adjuvant chemotherapy in locally advanced non-small-cell lung carcinoma (letter). *Journal of the National Cancer Institute* **8**: 58.

Lee YC, Luh SP, Wu RM, Lee CJ (1994) Adjuvant immunotherapy with intrapleural *Streptococcus pyogenes* (OK-432) in lung cancer patients after resection. *Cancer Immunology and Immunotherapy* **39**: 269–274.

Ludwig Lung Cancer Study Group (1985) Adverse effect of intrapleural *Corynebacterium parvae* as adjuvant therapy in stage I and II non-small cell carcinoma of lung. *Journal of Thoracic and Cardiovascular Surgery* **89**: 842.

Lung Cancer Study Group (1987) Effects of postoperative mediastinal radiation on completely resected stage II and stage III epidermoid cancer of the lung. *New England Journal of Medicine* **315**: 1377–1381.

Mattson K, Holsti LP, Holsti P et al. (1988) Inoperable NSCLC: radiation with or without chemotherapy. *European Journal of Cancer and Clinical Oncology* **24**: 477–82.

Mattson K, Ten Velde G, Krofta K, Cour-Chabernaud V, Abratt R (2000) Early results of an international phase III study evaluating Taxotere as neo-adjuvant therapy for radically treatable stage III NSCLC. *Lung Cancer* **29**(suppl 1): 90 (abstract 295).

Miller VA, Johnson D, Heelan RT et al. (2001) A pilot trial demonstrates the safety of ZD1839 (Iressa), an oral epidermal growth factor receptor tyrosine kinase inhibitor, in combination with carboplatin and paclitaxel in previously untreated advanced non-small cell lung cancer. *Proceedings of the American Society of Clinical Oncology* **20**: 326 (abstract 1301).

Morsac B, Scott C, Curran W (2001) A quality-adjusted time without symptoms and toxicity (QTWIST) analysis of Radiotherapy Oncology Group (RTOG). *Proceedings of the American Society of Clinical Oncology* **20**: 313a (abstract).

Morton RF, Jett JR, McGinnis WL et al. (1991) Thoracic radiation therapy alone compared with chemotherapy for locally unresectable non-small-cell carcinoma of the lung. *Annals of Internal Medicine* **115**: 681–686.

Mountain CF (1997) Revisions in the International System for Staging Lung Cancer. *Chest* **111**: 1710–1717.

National Institute for Clinical Excellence (2001) *Guidance on the Use of Docetaxel, Paclitaxel, Gemcitabine and Vinorelbine for the Treatment of Non-small Cell Lung Cancer.* London: NHS Executive.

Niiranen A, Niitamo-Korhonen S, Kouri M, Assendelft A, Mattson K, Pyrhonen S (1992) Adjuvant chemotherapy after radical surgery for non-small cell lung cancer: a randomised study. *Journal of Clinical Oncology* **10**: 1927–1932.

NSCLC Collaborative Group (1995) Chemotherapy in non-small cell lung cancer: a meta-analysis using updated data on individual patients from 52 randomised clinical trials. *British Medical Journal* **311**: 899–909.

Pantel K, Izbicki J, Passlick B et al. (1996) Frequency and prognostic significance of isolated tumour cells in bone marrow of patients with non-small cell lung cancer without overt metastasis. *The Lancet* **347**: 649–653.

Parkin DM, Pisani P, Ferlag J et al. (1999) Cancer statistics 1999. *CA: A Cancer Journal for Clinicians* **49**: 33–64.

Pass HI, Pogrebniak HW, Steinberg SM, Mulshine J, Minna JD (1992) Randomised trial of neoadjuvant therapy for lung cancer: interim analysis. *Annals of Thoracic Surgery* **53**: 9920–9998.

Pastorino U (1996) Benefits of neoadjuvant chemotherapy in NSCLC. *Chest* **109**: 96S–101S.

Perez-Soler R, Chachoua A, Huberman M et al. (2001) A phase II trial of the epidermal growth factor receptor (EGFR) tyrosine kinase inhibitor OSI-774, following platinum-based chemotherapy, in patients with advanced, EGFR-expressing non-small cell lung cancer. *Proceedings of the American Society of Clinical Oncology* **20**: 310 (abstract 1235).

Pisters KM (2000) The role of chemotherapy in early stage (stage I + II) resectable NSCLC. *Seminars for Radiation Oncology* **10**: 274–279.

PORT Meta-analysis Trialists Group (1998) Postoperative radiotherapy in non-small cell lung cancer: a systematic review and meta-analysis of individual patient data from nine randomised trials. *The Lancet* **352**: 257–263.

Rose PG, Bundy BN, Watkins EB et al. (1999) Concurrent cisplatin based radiotherapy and chemotherapy for locally advanced cervical cancer. *New England Journal of Medicine* **340**: 1144–1153.

Rosell R (1999) New approaches in the adjuvant and neoadjuvant therapy of NSCLC, including docetaxel (Taxotere) combinations. *Seminars in Oncology* **26**(suppl 11): 32–37.

Rosell R, Gomez-Codina J, Camps C et al. (1994) A Randomised trial comparing preoperative chemotherapy plus surgery with surgery alone in patients with non-small cell lung cancer. *New England Journal of Medicine* **330**: 153–158.

Rosell R, Gomez-Codina J, Camps C et al. (1999) Preresectional chemotherapy in stage IIIA non-small cell lung cancer: a 7-year assessment of a randomized controlled trial. *Lung Cancer* **47**: 7–14.

Roth JA, Fosella F, Komaki P et al. (1994) A randomised trial comparing preoperative chemotherapy and surgery with surgery alone in resectable stage IIIA NSCLC. *Journal of the National Cancer Institute* **86**: 673–680.

Roth JA, Atkinson EN, Fosella F et al. (1998) Long term follow up of patients enrolled in a randomised trial comparing perioperative chemotherapy and surgery with surgery alone in resectable stage IIIA non small cell lung cancer. *Lung Cancer* **21**: 1–6.

Rowell NP, Williams CJ (2001) Radical radiotherapy for stage I/II NSCLC in patients not sufficiently fit for or declining surgery (medically inoperable) (Cochrane Review). The Cochrane Library, Issue 3, Oxford.

Royal College of Radiologists' Clinical Information Network (1999) Guidelines on the non-surgical management of lung cancer. *Clinical Oncology* **11**: S23–S28.

Saunders M, Dische S, Barrett A et al. on behalf of the CHART Steering Committee (1999) Continuous hyperfractionated accelerated radiotherapy versus conventional radiotherapy in NSCLC: mature data from the randomised multi-centre trial. *Radiotherapeutic Oncology* **52**: 137–148.

Sause W, Scott C, Taylor S et al. (1995) RTOG 88–08, ECOG 4588, preliminary results of a phase III trial in regionally advanced, unresectable non-small cell lung cancer. *Journal of the National Cancer Institute* **87**: 189–205.

Sause W, Kolesar P, Taylor S et al. (2000) Final results of phase III trial in regionally advanced unresectable non-small cell lung cancer. *Chest* **117**: 358–64.

Schaake-Koning C, van den Bogaert W, Dalesio O et al. (1992) Effects of concomitant cisplatin and radiotherapy on inoperable non-small cell lung cancer. *New England Journal of Medicine* **326**: 524–30.

Sculier JP, Paesmans M, Lafitte JJ et al. (1999) A randomised phase III trial comparing consolidation treatment with further chemotherapy to chest irradiation in patients with initially unresectable locoregional non-small-cell lung cancer responding to induction chemotherapy. *Annals in Oncology* **10**: 295–303.

Shepherd FA (1997) Alternatives to chemotherapy and radiotherapy as adjuvant treatment for lung cancer. *Lung Cancer* **17**(suppl 1): S121–S136.

Siegenthaler MP, Pisters KM, Merriman KW et al. (2001) Preoperative chemotherapy does not increase surgical morbididty. *Annals of Thoracic Surgery* **71**: 1105–1112.

Takita H, Hollinshead AC, Adler RH et al. (1991) Adjuvant, specific, active immunotherapy for resectable squamous cell lung carcinoma: a 5-year survival analysis. *Journal of Surgical Oncology* **46**: 9–14.

Trovo NG, Minotel E, Fravelun G et al. (1992) Radiotherapy versus radiotherapy enhanced by cisplatin in stage III non-small cell lung cancer. *International Journal of Radiation Oncology, Biology and Physics* **24**: 11–16.

Trovo NG, Minotel E, Veronesi A et al. (1990) Combined radiotherapy and chemotherapy versus radiotherapy alone in locally-advanced epidermoid bronchogenic carcinoma. A randomised study. *Cancer* **65**: 400–404.

Whyte RI, Schork MA, Sloan H, Orringer MB, Kirsh MM (1992) Adjuvant treatment using transfer-factor for bronchogenic-carcinoma – long-term follow-up. *Annals of Thoracic Surgery* **53**: 391–396.

Wolf M, Muller H, Siefart U et al. (2001) Randomised phase III trial of adjuvant radiotherapy versus adjuvant chemotherapy followed by radiotherapy in patients with N2 positive non-small cell lung cancer. *Proceedings of the American Society of Clinical Oncology* **20**: abstract 1242.

Chapter 6

An update of the evidence on chemotherapy in advanced or metastatic NSCLC

David Gibbs, Mary O'Brien and Andreas Polychronis

Non-small cell lung cancer (NSCLC) is a major health problem. It accounts for 80% of all primary lung cancers and is the most common cancer-related cause of death in men and the second most common cancer-related cause of death in women in the European Union (Levi et al. 1999). Over 60% of cases present with advanced (stage IIIB or IV) disease and, in this group, prognosis is poor. The 1-year survival rate is 10–20% and fewer than 1% of patients are alive at 5 years (Non-small Cell Lung Cancer Collaborative Group 2001).

An important development in the management of patients with advanced NSCLC is the recognition that treatment with palliative chemotherapy confers a modest improvement in survival and has a beneficial effect on the symptoms of advanced disease and global quality of life. This chapter discusses some of the trials on which these conclusions are based, considers the evidence supporting the different regimens available and outlines current directions of research.

First-line chemotherapy
Chemotherapy compared with best supportive care

The Non-small Cell Lung Cancer Collaborative Group (2001) performed a meta-analysis of the randomised trials of chemotherapy in NSCLC. The meta-analysis was last updated in February 2000 and a new revision was published in 2001. Included in the analysis were 11 trials containing 1190 patients comparing chemotherapy with best supportive care in patients with advanced disease. The authors noted substantial variation in trial design, conduct and agents used, e.g. one trial included only patients with metastatic disease, whereas the others included patients with both locally advanced and metastatic disease. Two trials used long-term alkylating agents and one used single-agent etoposide. The remaining eight trials used cisplatin-based chemotherapy, seven of which used a combination of cisplatin and vinca alkaloids or etoposide. The cisplatin dose ranged from 40 mg/m^2 to 120 mg/m^2 per cycle. Despite the heterogeneity resulting from the differences in study design, pooled results from the cisplatin-containing trials showed a clear benefit in favour of chemotherapy with a hazard ratio of 0.73 for death *(p < 0.0001, a 27% reduction in the risk of death)*. This is equivalent to an absolute improvement in survival of 10% at 1 year, improving survival from 15% to 25%, or an improvement in median survival of 1.5 months, improving median survival from 4 months to 5.5 months.

A subgroup analysis was performed to determine whether any particular groups benefited more or less from chemotherapy. There was no evidence that any group of patients specified by age, sex, histological cell type, performance status or stage benefited more or less from chemotherapy. This may reflect the highly selected nature of patients on clinical trials because there is case series evidence that patients with poor performance status (ECOG ≤ 3) have high early mortality from chemotherapy and may gain less benefit (Hickish et al. 1995). We have updated our previous data on performance status, toxicity, response rate and survival (Table 6.1 and Figure 6.1) and currently recommend strongly that patients with performance status 3 should not be treated and those with performance status 2 should have the risks and benefits carefully explained.

Table 6.1 Performance status and outcome in patients receiving chemotherapy for NSCLC

Performance status	0/1	2	3/4
n	523	224	48
6 months survival (%)	66	45	13
1 year survival (%)	34	18	3
Response rate (%)	35	27	13

Single-agent chemotherapy compared with best supportive care

Several phase III trials comparing single-agent 'third-generation' agents with best supportive care in first-line chemotherapy have been published since the last update of the meta-analysis and are summarised in Table 6.2.

Some 157 patients with stage IIIB and IV disease received either paclitaxel 200 mg/m^2 every 3 weeks with best supportive care or best supportive care alone. Patients receiving best supportive care were able to have radiotherapy, corticosteroids, antibiotics, analgesics, antiemetics, transfusions and other symptomatic therapy as required. The median survival in the paclitaxel group was 6.8 months, compared with 4.8 months in the best supportive care group ($p = 0.037$). Global quality of life (QoL) was the same in both arms of the trial except for a subgroup in the QoL index that favoured the paclitaxel arm. Although fewer patients in the paclitaxel group required radiotherapy, more required hospitalisation during the study (58% vs 41%), possibly because of their longer survival and thus time on study (Ranson et al. 2000).

Of patients with locally advanced or metastatic disease, 300 were randomised to receive best supportive care or best supportive care and gemcitabine 1000 mg/m^2 on days 1, 8 and 15 of a 28-day cycle. Unlike other studies, the primary endpoints were

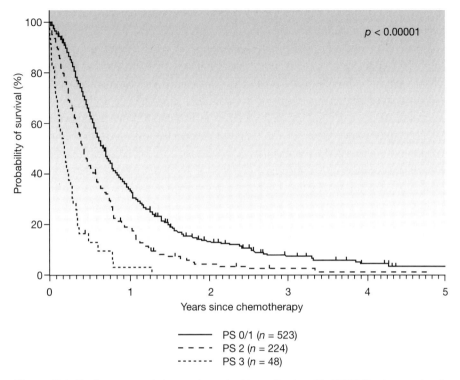

Figure 6.1 Performance status and survival in patients with NSCLC who received chemotherapy

Table 6.2 Trials comparing third-generation agents with best supportive care

Regimen	Number	Response rate (%)	Median survival (weeks)	Reference
Paclitaxel	157	16	**29**	Ranson et al. (2000)
BSC			**21**	
Vinorelbine	191	20	**28**	Elderly Lung Cancer
BSC			**21**	Vinorelbine Italian Study Group (1999)
Docetaxel	207	13	**26**[a]	Roszkowski et al. (2000)
BSC			**24**	
Gemcitabine	300	19	24	Anderson et al. (2000)[b]
BSC			25	

Figures in bold face indicate a significant ($p < 0.05$) difference between groups; BSC, best supportive care; N/A, not available.
[a]1-year survival favours chemotherapy. [b]Study not powered for survival.

QoL measures. They were defined as the percentage change in mean SS14 score (14 question symptom score) between baseline and 2 months, and the proportion of patients with a marked (≥ 25%) improvement in SS14 score sustained for 4 weeks or more. The response rate in the gemcitabine group was 19% and patients in this group were significantly more likely to experience a sustained improvement in QoL scores than patients receiving best supportive care alone. However, the authors noted that only one-fifth to one-third of trial patients gained relief from common disease-related symptoms such as chest pain, cough and dyspnoea. In contrast, the requirement for palliative radiotherapy was significantly delayed in the gemcitabine-treated group (29 weeks vs. 4 weeks). No difference in survival was noted between the groups (5.7 months on gemcitabine and best supportive care, 5.9 months on best supportive care alone, $p = 0.84$; Anderson et al. 2000), although this study was not powered to detect a difference in survival.

Of patients with unresectable or metastatic disease and performance status 0–1, 207 were randomised to receive either best supportive care (BSC) alone (71 patients) or BSC with docetaxel 100 mg/m^2 every 21 days (137 patients). The response rate to chemotherapy was 13%. Median survival was 6 months in the docetaxel arm and 5.7 months in the BSC-alone arm. However, the 2-year survival rate was significantly longer in the docetaxel arm than in the BSC-alone arm (12% vs 0%). QoL (assessed by the EORTC QLQ-C30 questionnaire) was improved in the docetaxel arm over the BSC-alone arm. In the docetaxel group there was less use of analgesics and palliative radiotherapy and improvement in dyspnoea and pain, but not in haemoptysis or cough. Of the docetaxel group, 51% required hospitalisation compared with 30% of the BSC arm (Roszkowski et al. 2000).

These recent studies confirm that active single-agent chemotherapy results in improved quality of life in patients with advanced NSCLC and a small improvement in overall survival. It is of interest that chemotherapy was associated with a decrease in the need for palliative radiotherapy, but this may result in more hospitalisation in some cases although less in others. These are important issues that need to be addressed in future studies.

Best standard of care

The evidence that chemotherapy is superior to BSC alone is relatively clear. However, there is less evidence to support the use of any one particular regimen over another, at least in terms of efficacy.

The role of cisplatin

Cisplatin has been considered a mainstay of chemotherapy in NSCLC, although individual trials provide little evidence to support this belief. Trials comparing platinum-containing with non-platinum-containing chemotherapy generally, but not always, showed that the addition of platinum increases response rate, with few showing an increase in survival associated with platinum (Harvey et al. 1987; Rosso et al. 1988; Veeder et al. 1992; Gridelli et al. 1996; Splinter et al. 1996; Buccheri and Ferrigno 1997). However, a meta-analysis of trials conducted in the USA between 1973 and 1994 showed that patients treated with platinum-containing chemotherapy had a median survival of 6 months, compared with 4.7 months in patients treated with non-platinum-containing regimens (Breathnach et al. 2001). None of the non-platinum treatments in this meta-analysis included gemcitabine, taxanes or vinorelbine, so these survival differences may not apply to modern regimens as suggested by the trials comparing gemcitabine with cisplatin–etoposide, all of which show equivalent activity (Manegold et al. 1997; Perng et al. 1997; ten Bokkel Huinink et al. 1999). The addition of cisplatin to active single agents appears to result in a trend to increased response rate, but this does not result in an increase in survival (Table 6.3).

Table 6.3 Trials comparing single third-generation agents with platinum-containing doublets

Regimen	Number	Response rate (%)	Median survival (weeks)	Reference
Gemcitabine	72	6	42	Berardi et al.
Gemcitabine–cisplatin		24	42	(2001)
Vinorelbine	231	**16**	33	Depierre et al.
Vinorelbine–cisplatin		**43**	32	(1994)
Gemcitabine	332	12	40	Sederholm
Gemcitabine–carboplatin		30	44	(2002)
Docetaxel	307	18	40	Georgoulias et al.
Docetaxel-cisplatin		**35**	52	(2002)

Figures in bold face indicate a significant ($p < 0.05$) difference between groups; N/A, not available.

Four trials examined the effects of the addition of other active agents to single-agent cisplatin and are summarised in Table 6.4. Three trials (comparing cisplatin with cisplatin–vindesine, cisplatin–vinorelbine and cisplatin–gemcitabine) showed improved response rates for combination over single-agent therapy. The addition of gemcitabine or vinorelbine increased survival over single-agent cisplatin. It is important to note that only the three latest trials had sufficient power to detect a 2-month difference in median survival. Generally speaking, haematological toxicity was greater in the combination arms than in the cisplatin-alone arms; otherwise toxicity was comparable. In the two trials to include QoL measurements, there was no difference in quality of life between the regimens (Gatzemeier et al. 2000; Sandler et al. 2000).

Several trials have examined the effect of cisplatin dose or dose intensity on outcome. A trial comparing vindesine and cisplatin 80 mg/m^2 or 120 mg/m^2 in 85 patients showed that the higher-dose cisplatin resulted in increased median survival (93 vs 43 weeks, $p = 0.02$) (Gralla et al. 1981). Subsequent trials comparing cisplatin 50 mg/m^2 and 100 mg/m^2 (Gandara et al. 1993), cisplatin 105 mg/m^2 3 versus 4-weekly (Font et al. 1999) showed no relationship between cisplatin dose and outcome.

Table 6.4 Trials comparing single-agent cisplatin with cisplatin doublets

Regimen	Number	Response rate (%)	Median survival (weeks)	Reference
Cisplatin	160	**12**	39	Kawahara et al. (1991)
Vindesine–cisplatin		**29**	45	
Cisplatin	432	**12**	**26**	Wozniak et al. (1998)
Vinorelbine–cisplatin		**26**	**34**	
Cisplatin	414	17	37	Gatzemeier et al.
Cisplatin–paclitaxel		26	35	(2000)
Cisplatin	522	**11**	**33**	Sandler et al. (2000)
Gemcitabine–cisplatin		**30**	**39**	

Figures in bold face indicate a significant ($p < .05$) difference between groups; N/A, not available.

Taken together, these data suggest that cisplatin has single-agent activity in NSCLC and, combined with new agents, the response rate is improved. However, the combinations are more toxic and we need more data on survival benefits in advanced disease. The optimum dose of cisplatin remains to be determined.

The role of carboplatin

The relative efficacy of carboplatin compared with cisplatin in lung cancer has not been well established, although many investigators believe them to be equivalent. A multiple-arm randomised trial comparing treatment with mitomycin–vinblastine–cisplatin (MVP) or single-agent carboplatin showed a response rate of 9% with carboplatin compared with 20% for MVP. Despite this, there was a trend to improved overall survival favouring carboplatin (Bonomi et al. 1989). In a trial comparing cisplatin–etoposide with carboplatin–etoposide, the response rates (25%, 20%) and median survivals (25 weeks, 24 weeks) were equivalent (Klastersky et al. 1990). A trial comparing cisplatin–paclitaxel with carboplatin–paclitaxel has been published in abstract, and preliminary data suggest that the two regimens are equivalent in activity (Macha et al. 1998). A three-arm trial in 1220 patients comparing docetaxel-cisplatin to vinorelbine-cisplatin or docetaxel-carboplatin to vinorelbine-cisplatin demonstrated for the first time a significantly longer survival of one platinum doublet over a standard regimen. For docetaxel-cisplatin versus vinorelbine-cisplatin the median survival was 11.3 months versus 10.1 months ($p = 0.044$) and the 2-year survival was also significantly different (21% vs 14%). Survival and response rates for docetaxel-carboplatin were similar to those of vinorelbine-cisplatin. Quality of life was consistently superior for both docetaxel arms compared to the control arm (Rodriguez et al. 2001). A study recently published compared mitomycin C with vindesine and either cisplatin 120 mg/m^2 or carboplatin 500 mg/m^2 in 221 patients and reported a significantly improved progression-free survival ($p = 0.005$) and survival ($p = 0.008$) in the carboplatin-treated patients (Jelic et al. 2001).

Combination chemotherapy

Combination chemotherapy offers the possibility of improved outcome through non-cross-resistance or true synergy. Trials have tested several combination strategies, including two-drug regimens (doublets) and three-drug regimens (triplets).

Trials comparing platinum-containing doublets

A number of trials comparing doublets have been performed (Table 6.5). In two trials, one comparing cisplatin–vinblastine with carboplatin–gemcitabine (Grigorescu et al. 2000) and the other comparing carboplatin–paclitaxel with cisplatin–etoposide, a significant difference survival was noted (Bonomi et al. 1997). However, a trial comparing carboplatin–paclitaxel with cisplatin–vinorelbine showed no difference between the two regimens in terms of response rate, quality of life or survival (Kelly et al. 2001). Leucopenia was more common in the vinorelbine–cisplatin arm than the carboplatin–paclitaxel arm, and neuropathy more common in the latter arm. There were more discontinuations as a result of toxicity in the vinorelbine–cisplatin arm, but costs were significantly higher in the carboplatin–paclitaxel arm. Cisplatin–gemcitabine, carboplatin–paclitaxel and cisplatin–vinorelbine are being compared in 612 patients. Preliminary toxicity data show that leucopenia occurs more frequently in the cisplatin–vinorelbine group and thrombocytopenia in the cisplatin–gemcitabine arm. Response and survival data show no difference between the three treatments (Scagliotti et al. 2001). These trials suggest that various doublets have equivalent activity and differ mainly in the type of toxicity that they produce, rather than its severity. A meta-analysis of trials comparing second to third generation chemotherapy suggests that third generation regimens increase response rate by approximately 13% and 1-year survival by 4% compared with second generation regimens (Baggstrom et al. 2002). In summary, it is our opinion that all the new third-generation doublets are superior to the second-generation doublet, but that there is no obvious superior combination.

Trials comparing platinum-containing doublets and triplets

Current phase III trials are concentrating on the combination of two or more active agents, either as triplets or as sequential doublets. Such sequential regimens have the theoretical advantage of allowing the administration of higher dose intensities of individual agents than is possible when three or four drugs are given simultaneously. Recent trials are summarized in Table 6.6. Preliminary results suggest that third-generation triple-drug regimens may increase response rates and that this may be associated with an increase in median survival. However, these data are early and do not suggest that there should be a change in practice yet.

Table 6.5 Trials comparing chemotherapy doublets

Regimen	Number	Response rate (%)	Median survival (weeks)	Reference
Cisplatin–vinblastine	110	**4**	**38**	Grigorescu et al.
Carboplatin–gemcitabine		**21**	**46**	(2000)
Etoposide–cisplatin	135	**22**	31	Cardenal et al.
Gemcitabine–cisplatin		**41**	37	(1999)
Epirubicin–cisplatin	228	33	45	Martoni et al.
Vinorelbine–cisplatin		27	41	(1998)
Carboplatin–paclitaxel	329	29	45	Kosmidis et al.
Gemcitabine–paclitaxel		36	53	(2000)
Paclitaxel–cisplatin	332	**41**	42	Giaccone et al.
Tenoposide–cisplatin		**28**	41	(1998)
Etoposide–cisplatin	369	14	N/A	Belani et al.
Paclitaxel–carboplatin		21		(1998)
Docetaxel–cisplatin	441	32	N/A	Georgoulias et al.
Docetaxel–gemcitabine		31		(2001)
Etoposide–cisplatin	574	13	33	Bonomi et al.
Carboplatin–paclitaxel		25*	41*	(1997)
Carboplatin–paclitaxel + GCSF		28*	46*	
Docetaxel–carboplatin	1218	23.9	37.6	Fossella et al.
Docetaxel–cisplatin		31.6	**45.2**	ECCO-11 (2001)
Vinorelbine–cisplatin		24.5	40.4	Abst # 562
Cisplatin–paclitaxel	1207	21	32	Schiller et al.
Cisplatin–gemcitabine		22	33	(2002)
Cisplatin–docetaxel		17	30	
Carboplatin–paclitaxel		17	33	

Figures in bold face indicate a significant ($p < 0.05$) difference between groups; GCSF, granulocyte colony-stimulating factor; N/A, not available.

*Significantly greater than etoposide-cisplatin doublet.

Table 6.6 Trials comparing chemotherapy doublets and triplets

Regimen	Number	Response rate (%)	Median survival (weeks)	Reference
Carboplatin–paclitaxel	71	**28**	33	Hussein et al.
Carboplatin–paclitaxel–gemcitabine		**61**	45	(2000)
Mitomycin–ifosfamide–cisplatin	179	37	46	Depierre et al.
Mitomycin–ifosfamide–cisplatin → vinorelbine		37	55	(2001)
Cisplatin–gemcitabine–vinorelbine	180	47	**51**	Comella et al.
Gemcitabine–cisplatin		37	**42**	(2000)
Vinorelbine–cisplatin		25	35	
Carboplatin–gemcitabine → paclitaxel	204	21	36	Edelman et al.
Carboplatin–vinorelbine → docetaxel		28	36	(2001)
Mitomycin–vinblastine–cisplatin or	232	33	N/A	Danson et al.
Mitomycin–ifosfamide–cisplatin				(2001)
Gemcitabine–cisplatin		39		
Carboplatin–paclitaxel–gemcitabine	243	34	44	Thompson
Carboplatin–paclitaxel–vinorelbine		42	21	et al. (2001)
Paclitaxel–gemcitabine		29	33	
Paclitaxel–vinorelbine		29	30	
Mitomycin–vinblastine–cisplatin	247	41	17	Gebbia et al.
Vinorelbine–cisplatin		38	18	(2002)
Mitomycin–vinblastine–cisplatin	248	27	27	Melo et al.
Vinorelbine–cisplatin		**37**	**38**	(2002)
Gemcitabine–cisplatin		**48**	**41**	
Mitomycin–ifosfamide–cisplatin	307	**26**	41	Crino et al.
Gemcitabine–cisplatin		**38**	37	(1999)
Cisplatin–gemcitabine–vinorelbine	343	**44**	**51**	Comella
Cisplatin–gemcitabine		28	38	(2001)
Cisplatin–gemcitabine–paclitaxel		**48**	**51**	
Gemcitabine–cisplatin	562	41	41	Alberola et al.
Gemcitabine–cisplatin–vinorelbine		40	34	(2001)
Gemcitabine–vinorelbine → Ifosfamide–vinorelbine		24	45	

Figures in bold face indicate a significant ($p < 0.05$) difference between groups,
N/A: not available. Arrows indicate sequential administration.

Non-platinum combination chemotherapy with third-generation agents

The growing evidence for the equal efficacy of third-generation agents and platinum have led to trials of non-platinum-containing combination therapy. A trial comparing gemcitabine–vinorelbine with vinorelbine in patients aged over 70 with advanced disease showed a significantly higher response rate (22% and 15%) and median survival (29 weeks and 18 weeks) for the combination arm. Importantly, patients noted a greater improvement in dyspnoea and cough in the combination arm. However, there was significant toxicity in both groups, and almost half the patients experienced severe fatigue, anorexia or constipation.

Patients with poor performance status and medical co-morbidity were more likely to have severe toxicity requiring treatment cessation (Frasci et al. 2000). A subsequent trial comparing single-agent gemcitabine or vinorelbine with the combination in 700 patients showed no benefit from the chemotherapy combination (Gridelli et al. 2001).

Some 441 patients with advanced NSCLC received either cisplatin–docetaxel or gemcitabine–docetaxel. There was no difference in response rate (35% and 32%) or median survival (10 months and 9.5 months) between the groups. Measures of toxicity favoured non-platinum therapy with regard to nausea, vomiting and peripheral neuropathy. Non-platinum therapy resulted in more neutropenia and oedema (Georgoulias et al. 2001). Preliminary results are also available for a trial that randomised 480 patients among cisplatin–paclitaxel, cisplatin–gemcitabine and paclitaxel–gemcitabine. Less grade 3/4 vomiting, thrombocytopenia and sensory neuropathy occurred in the paclitaxel–gemcitabine group; in other respects, toxicities were similar (Van Meerbeeck et al. 2001).

Duration of therapy

There is uncertainty surrounding the optimal duration of therapy for advanced NSCLC. Current recommendations range from two to three courses of chemotherapy, to continuation of treatment until disease progression. A recent trial addressed this question in patients receiving MVP chemotherapy for advanced NSCLC. Before the start of treatment, patients were randomly assigned to receive either three or six cycles of chemotherapy. In the patients assigned to six cycles, 73% completed three cycles but only 31% completed six cycles. Radiological response rate, symptomatic response rate, survival and time to progression were equivalent among the groups. Patients who were assigned to continuing chemotherapy had significantly increased fatigue and a trend to increased nausea and vomiting. Patients assigned to three courses tended to have improved global health, physical function and emotional well-being (Smith et al. 2001); 230 patients were randomized between carboplatin–paclitaxel 3-weekly for four cycles or continued until disease progression. The overall response rate was 21% and median survival for all patients was 33 weeks, with no difference observed between the groups (Socinski et al. 2001). It is important to note that the median number of courses was four in both groups.

Choosing between regimens: a health economic analysis

The Ottawa Regional Cancer Centre has produced a decision framework for chemotherapy in advanced NSCLC, incorporating a cost-effectiveness analysis. The model incorporated costs from healthcare utilisation for non-cancer causes, costs related to initial diagnosis and staging, chemotherapy, radiotherapy, palliative care and finally terminal care. Included within the model were estimates of gain in survival and estimates of the utility values of various chemotherapy regimens, determined in a survey of 24 oncologists involved in the treatment of lung cancer. The regimens included in the model were cisplatin–vinblastine, cisplatin–etoposide, cisplatin–vinorelbine, single-agent gemcitabine, single-agent vinorelbine and cisplatin–paclitaxel.

Using this model, cisplatin–vinblastine resulted in a cost saving over BSC and was the most cost-effective regimen overall. Single-agent vinorelbine and cisplatin–vinorelbine were the next most effective regimens. Using an alternative analysis, chemotherapy regimens were compared against a threshold cost for years of life gained. At a threshold cost of $US50 000, which is considered to be a reasonable cost compared with other medical interventions, cisplatin–vinorelbine was the most effective and single-agent gemcitabine was ranked second. If cost per quality year-adjusted life-year (QUALY) was considered, single-agent gemcitabine was the most effective regimen, largely because of the greater utility assigned to it by oncologists.

Although this conclusion was drawn using data from the Canadian population, the method can probably be generalised to other populations and may provide a way to choose between regimens, at least on a national consensus basis (Berthelot et al. 2000).

Further evidence supporting the use of gemcitabine alone or in combination with cisplatin is derived from the work of Lees and co-workers (2002) showing these regimens to be cost-effective therapies when compared with best supportive care and standard or novel chemotherapy combinations. These authors are convinced that chemotherapy regimens containing gemcitabine therefore represent good value for money and efficient use of healthcare resources in the treatment of advanced NSCLC.

Second-line therapy

There are now two published trials showing that chemotherapy at relapse improves survival and quality of life. In a trial comparing docetaxel with BSC, patients were stratified by performance status and best response to cisplatin chemotherapy, and were then randomized to treatment with docetaxel 100 mg/m^2 (49 patients) or 75 mg/m^2 (55 patients) or BSC. The overall response rate was 5.8% but no responses were seen in patients who had progressed while on first-line chemotherapy. The median duration of survival for the chemotherapy arm was 7.0 months compared with 4.6 months for the BSC group; the 1-year survival rates for chemotherapy and

BSC were 29% and 19%, respectively. Eleven patients (22.4%) developed febrile neutropenia (three fatal cases) at the higher docetaxel dose, compared with only one patient (1.8%) at the lower dose (no fatal cases). As a result, the high-dose arm was closed prematurely. Measures of QoL favoured chemotherapy; there was significantly less fatigue and pain in this group and less use of analgesics and radiotherapy (Shepherd et al. 2000). Of patients with relapsed or refractory disease, 373 were randomised to receive docetaxel 75 mg/m^2, docetaxel 100 mg/m^2 or vinorelbine or ifosfamide. Response rates (7%, 11%) favoured the two docetaxel groups over vinorelbine or ifosfamide (0.8%). Time to progression and progression-free survival favoured docetaxel, but overall survival did not differ between the treatment arms (Fossella et al. 2000).

Paclitaxel and gemcitabine have been assessed as treatment at relapse in phase II trials, but not yet in phase III. The role of combination treatment has not been adequately explored, nor has the use of salvage treatment in patients who have received gemcitabine or taxanes as first-line treatment. Nevertheless, these studies provide evidence for the benefit of second-line docetaxel in selected patients with relapsed disease. Although objective responses are not seen in patients with platinum-resistant disease, it is possible that these patients experienced a gain in survival. The role of salvage therapy in this group needs further investigation.

New strategies

Current regimens and strategies in advanced NSCLC have provided modest improvements in survival and quality of life. Further improvements are unlikely to come without the identification of new targets for therapy. The following is a brief outline of some of the strategies being pursued.

Phase II studies with conventional cytotoxic agents

Most of the current work in this area is on the testing of new combinations and schedules of existing agents, e.g. a randomised phase II study shows comparable activity and toxicity between docetaxel–cisplatin and docetaxel–irinotecan (Takeda et al. 2000). Some new agents are being assessed in advanced NSCLC. Temozolomide (Adonizio et al. 2001), a novel dihydrofolate reductase inhibitor (Azzoli et al. 2001), a platinum analogue, ZD0473 (Treat et al. 2001), an oral 5-fluorouracil (5FU) analogue, S-1 (Niitani et al. 2000), and a topoisomerase I inhibitor, exactecan (Talbot et al. 2000), all show evidence of modest activity in phase II trials.

Novel strategies

A number of novel strategies that showed promise in phase I/II evaluation are being tested in phase III trials (http://cancernet.nci.nih.gov/trialsrch.shtml). They include bevacizumab (anti-vascular endothelial growth factor antibody) in combination with carboplatin–paclitaxel, ZD1839 (epidermal growth factor receptor [EGFR]-associated tyrosine kinase inhibitor – Baselga et al. 2000) in combination with carboplatin–paclitaxel, and exisulind (cGMP phosphodiesterase inhibitor – Thompson et al. 2000) in combination with docetaxel in patients with relapsed NSCLC. HER-2/neu is expressed in 20–50% of NSCLC and the successful addition of trastuzumab (anti-HER-2/neu monoclonal antibody) to chemotherapy in metastatic breast cancer has led to its trial in NSCLC. Phase II trials show that it can be administered in conjunction with carboplatin–paclitaxel in advanced NCSLC (Langer et al. 2001). The addition of anti-sense modulators of signalling cascades such as protein kinase C (Yuen et al. 2000) and *h*-ras (Dang et al. 2001) to carboplatin–paclitaxel are the subject of ongoing phase III trials.

Conclusions

There is a substantial body of evidence that patients with NSCLC may benefit from palliative chemotherapy, with a small increase in survival and a period of improved QoL. Despite a large number of clinical trials involving thousands of patients, there is no one regimen that is clearly superior to others in all respects. Platinum-based therapy is the *de facto* standard of care. Cisplatin in combination with vinorelbine, gemcitabine or paclitaxel are acceptable choices in patients with good performance status as reported by the National Institute for Clinical Excellence (NICE). However, in the UK, MVP and MIC (mitomycin, ifosfamide and cisplatin) will still be appropriate regimens for a percentage of our patients. Carboplatin-based regimens are attractive because they are more easily administered, but there have been fewer large trials of carboplatin-based regimens. Single-agent therapy with gemcitabine, vinorelbine or a taxane is a reasonable choice for patients who may not tolerate platinum-based therapy. Platinum-containing triplets, non-platinum doublets and sequential doublets remain investigational but may play a larger role in future.

There is evidence to support the use of second-line docetaxel in selected patients. The place of other active agents, singly or in combination, remains to be determined in this setting.

References

Adonizio C, Langer CJ, Huang C et al. (2001) Temozolomide in the treatment of advanced NSCLC: Phase II evaluation in previously treated patients. *Proceedings of the American Society of Clinical Oncology* **20**: abstract 1375.

Alberola, V, Camps C, Provencia M et al. (2001) Cisplatin/gemcitabine (CG) vs cisplatin/ gemcitabine/vinorelbine (CGV) vs sequential doublets of gemcitabine/vinorelbine followed by ifosfamide/vinorelbine (GV/IV) in advanced non-small cell lung cancer (NSCLC): Results of a Spanish Lung Cancer Group Phase III Trial (GEPC/98-02). *Proceedings of the American Society of Clinical Oncology* **20**: abstract 1229.

Anderson H, Hopwood P, Stephens R et al. (2000) Gemcitabine plus best supportive care (BSC) vs BSC in inoperable non-small cell lung cancer – a randomized trial with quality of life as the primary outcome. UK NSCLC Gemcitabine Group. *British Journal of Cancer* **83**: 447–453.

Azzoli C, Krug L, Miller V et al. (2001) Phase II study of 10-propargyl-10-deazaaminopterin (PDX) in previously-treated patients with advanced non-small cell lung cancer (NSCLC). *Proceedings of the American Society of Clinical Oncology* **20**: abstract 1321.

Baggstrom M, Socinski M, Hensing T et al. (2002) Third generation chemotherapy regimens improve survival over second generation regimens in stage IIIB/IV NSCLC: a meta-analysis of the published literature. *Proceedings of the American Society of Clinical Oncology* **21**: abstract 1222.

Baselga J, Herbst R, LoRusso P et al. (2000) Continuous administration of ZD1839 (Iressa), a novel oral epidermal growth factor receptor tyrosine kinase inhibitor (EGFR-TKI), in patients with five selected tumor types: evidence of activity and good tolerability. *Proceedings of the American Society of Clinical Oncology* **19**: abstract 686.

Belani CP, Natale RB, Lee JS et al. (1998) Randomized phase III trial comparing cisplatin/etoposide versus carboplatin/paclitaxel in advanced and metastatic non-small cell lung cancer (NSCLC). *Proceedings of the American Society of Clinical Oncology* **19**: abstract 1751.

Berardi R, Porfiri E, Massidda B et al. (2001) Gemcitabine (GEM) and cisplatin (PL) versus gemcitabine alone in stage IV non small cell lung cancer (NSCLC): Preliminary results of a randomized multicenter phase III study. *Proceedings of the American Society of Clinical Oncology* **20**: abstract 1385.

Berthelot J.-M, Will BP, Evans WK et al. (2000) Decision framework for chemotherapeutic interventions for metastatic non-small-cell lung cancer. *Journal of the National Cancer Institute* **92**: 1321–1329.

Bonomi P, Kim K, Kusler J et al. (1997) Cisplatin/etoposide vs paclitaxel/cisplatin/G-CSF vs paclitaxel/cisplatin in non-small-cell lung cancer. *Oncology (Huntington)* **11**(4 suppl 3): 9–10.

Bonomi PD, Finkelstein DM, Ruckdeschel JC et al. (1989) Combination chemotherapy versus single agents followed by combination chemotherapy in stage IV non-small-cell lung cancer: a study of the Eastern Cooperative Oncology Group. *Journal of Clinical Oncology* **7**: 1602–1613.

Breathnach OS, Freidlin B, Conley B et al. (2001) Twenty-two years of phase III trials for patients with advanced non- small-cell lung cancer: sobering results. *Journal of Clinical Oncology* **19**: 1734–1742.

Buccheri G, Ferrigno D (1997) Randomized trial of *cis*-platinum-based chemotherapy (MVP) versus non-platinum-based chemotherapy (MACC) in non-small cell lung cancer: a negative report from the Cuneo Lung Cancer Study Group (CuLCaSG). *Proceedings of the American Society of Clinical Oncology* **16**: abstract 1666.

Cardenal F, Lopez-Cabrerizo MP, Anton A et al. (1999) Randomized phase III study of gemcitabine-cisplatin versus etoposide- cisplatin in the treatment of locally advanced or metastatic non-small-cell lung cancer. *Journal of Clinical Oncology* **17**: 12–18.

Comella P (2001) Phase III trial of cisplatin/gemcitabine with or without vinorelbine or paclitaxel in advanced non-small cell lung cancer. *Seminars in Oncology* **28**(2 suppl 7): 7–10.

Comella P, Frasci G, Panza N et al. (2000) Randomized trial comparing cisplatin, gemcitabine, and vinorelbine with either cisplatin and gemcitabine or cisplatin and vinorelbine in advanced non-small-cell lung cancer: interim analysis of a phase III trial of the Southern Italy Cooperative Oncology Group. *Journal of Clinical Oncology* **18**: 1451–1457.

Crino L, Scagliotti GV, Ricci S et al. (1999) Gemcitabine and cisplatin versus mitomycin, ifosfamide, and cisplatin in advanced non-small-cell lung cancer: A randomized phase III study of the Italian Lung Cancer Project. *Journal of Clinical Oncology* **17**: 3522–3530.

Dang T, Johnson D, Kelly K et al. (2001) Multicenter phase II trial of an antisense inhibitor of H-ras (ISIS-2503) in advanced non-small cell lung cancer (NSCLC). *Proceedings of the American Society of Clinical Oncology* **20**: abstract 1325.

Danson S, Clemons M, Middleton M et al. (2001) A randomised study of gemcitabine with carboplatin (GC) versus mitomycin, vinblastine and cisplatin (MVP) or mitomycin C, ifosfamide and cisplatin (MIC) as first line chemotherapy in advanced non-small cell lung cancer (NSCLC). *Proceedings of the American Society of Clinical Oncology* **20**: abstract 1285.

Depierre A, Chastang C, Quoix E et al. (1994) Vinorelbine versus vinorelbine plus cisplatin in advanced non-small cell lung cancer: a randomized trial. *Annals of Oncology* **5**: 37–42.

Depierre A, Quoix E, Mercier M et al. (2001) Maintenance chemotherapy in advanced non-small cell lung cancer (NSCLC): a randomized study of vinorelbine (V) versus observation (OB) in patients (Pts) responding to induction therapy (French Cooperative Oncology Group). *Proceedings of the American Society of Clinical Oncology* **20**: abstract 1231.

Edelman M, Clark J, Chansky K et al. (2001) Randomized phase II Trial of sequential chemotherapy in advanced non-small cell lung cancer (SWOG 9806): carboplatin/gemcitabine (CARB/G) followed by paclitaxel (P) or cisplatin/vinorelbine (C/V) followed by docetaxel (D). *Proceedings of the American Society of Clinical Oncology* **20**: abstract 1254.

Elderly Lung Cancer Vinorelbine Italian Study Group (1999) Effects of vinorelbine on quality of life and survival of elderly patients with advanced non-small-cell lung cancer. The Elderly Lung Cancer Vinorelbine Italian Study Group. *Journal of the National Cancer Institute* **91**: 66–72.

Font A, Moyano AJ, Puerto JM et al. (1999) Increasing dose intensity of cisplatin-etoposide in advanced nonsmall cell lung carcinoma: a phase III randomized trial of the Spanish Lung Cancer Group. *Cancer* **85**: 855–863.

Fossella FV, DeVore R, Kerr RN et al. (2000) Randomized phase III trial of docetaxel versus vinorelbine or ifosfamide in patients with advanced non–small-cell lung cancer previously treated with platinum-containing chemotherapy regimens. *Journal of Clinical Oncology* **18**: 2354–2362.

Fossella FV (2001) Phase III study of taxotere and cisplatin (DC) or carboplatin (DCb) versus vinorelbine-cisplatin (DC) as first line therapy for advanced NSCLC. *European Journal of Cancer* **37**: 5154 (abstract 562).

Frasci G, Lorusso V, Panza N et al. (2000) Gemcitabine plus vinorelbine versus vinorelbine alone in elderly patients with advanced non-small-cell lung cancer. *Journal of Clinical Oncology* **18**: 2529–2536.

Gandara DR, Crowley J, Livingston RB et al. (1993) Evaluation of cisplatin intensity in metastatic non-small-cell lung cancer: a phase III study of the Southwest Oncology Group. *Journal of Clinical Oncology* **11**: 873–878.

Gatzemeier U, von Pawel J, Gottfried M et al. (2000) Phase III comparative study of high-dose cisplatin versus a combination of paclitaxel and cisplatin in patients with advanced non-small-cell lung cancer. *Journal of Clinical Oncology* **18**: 3390–3399.

Gebbia V, Galetta D, Riccardi F et al. (1998) Mitomycin C plus vindesine and cisplatin (MVP) versus vinorelbine and cisplatin (PV) in stage III - IV non-small cell lung cancer: a randomized phase III trial of the Southern Italy Oncology Study Groups (G.O.I.M). *Proceedings of the American Society of Clinical Oncology* **17**(Meeting Abstract).

Gebbia V, Galetta D, Riccardi F et al. (2002) Vinorelbine plus cisplatin versus cisplatin plus vindesine and mitomycin C in stage IIIB - IV non-small cell lung carcinoma: a prospective randomised study. *Lung Cancer* **37**(2): 179–187.

Georgoulias V, Papadakis E, Alexopoulos A et al. (2001) Platinum-based and non-platinum-based chemotherapy in advanced non-small-cell lung cancer: a randomised multicentre trial. *The Lancet* **357**: 1478–1484.

Georgoulias V, Ardavanis A, Agelidou M et al. (2002) Preliminary analysis of a multicentre phase III trial comparing docetaxel (D) versus docetaxel/cisplatin (DC) in patients with inoperable advanced and metastatic non-small cell lung cancer (NSCLC). *Proceedings of the Annual Meeting of the American Society of Clinical Oncology* **21**: abstract 1136.

Giaccone G, Splinter TA, Debruyne C et al. (1998) Randomized study of paclitaxel-cisplatin versus cisplatin-teniposide in patients with advanced non-small-cell lung cancer. The European Organization for Research and Treatment of Cancer Lung Cancer Cooperative Group. *Journal of Clinical Oncology* **16**: 2133–2141.

Gralla RJ, Casper ES, Kelsen DR et al. (1981) Cisplatin and vindesine combination chemotherapy for advanced carcinoma of the lung: A randomized trial investigating two dosage schedules. *Annals of Internal Medicine* **95**: 414–420.

Gridelli C, Perrone F, Gigolari S et al. (1996) Mitomycin C plus vindesine plus etoposide (MEV) versus mitomycin C plus vindesine plus cisplatin (MVP) in stage IV non-small-cell lung cancer: A phase III multicentre randomised trial. The Gruppo Oncologico Centro-Sud-Isole (G.O.C.S.I.). *Annals of Oncology* **7**: 821–826.

Gridelli C, Perrone F, Palmeri S et al. (2001) The MILES (Multicenter Italian Lung Cancer in the Elderly Study) phase III Trial: gemcitabine + vinorelbine vs vinorelbine and vs gemcitabine in elderly advanced NSCLC patients. *Proceedings of the American Society of Clinical Oncology* **20**: abstract 1230.

Grigorescu A, Draghici N, Gutulescu N et al. (2000) Gemcitabine plus carboplatin (GCB) versus cisplatin plus vinblastin (CV) in stage IIIB-IV non-small cell lung cancer (NSCLC). *Annals of Oncology* **11**(suppl 4).

Harvey VJ, Slevin ML, Cheek SP et al. (1987) A randomized trial comparing vindesine and cisplatinum to vindesine and methotrexate in advanced non small cell lung carcinoma. *European Journal of Cancer and Clinical Oncology* **23**: 1615–1619.

Hickish TF, Smith IE, Ashley S et al. (1995) Chemotherapy for elderly patients with lung cancer. *The Lancet* **346**: 580.

Hussein A, Birch R, Waller J et al. (2000) Preliminary results of a randomized study comparing paclitaxel and carboplatin (PC) with or without gemcitabine (G) in newly diagnosed non small cell lung cancer (NSCLC). *Proceedings of the American Society of Clinical Oncology* **19**: abstract 1973.

Jelic S, Mitrovic L, Radosavljevic D et al. (2001) Survival advantage for carboplatin substituting cisplatin in combination with vindesine and mitomycin C for stage IIIB and IV squamous-cell bronchogenic carcinoma: a randomised phase III study. *Lung Cancer* **34**: 1–13.

Kawahara M, Furuse K, Kodama N et al. (1991) A randomized study of cisplatin versus cisplatin plus vindesine for non-small cell lung carcinoma. *Cancer* **68**: 714–719.

Kawahara M, Furuse K, Segawa Y et al. (2001) Phase II study of S-1, a novel oral fluorouracil, in advanced non-small-cell lung cancer. *British Journal of Cancer* **85**(7): 939–943.

Kelly K, Crowley J, Bunn PA et al. (2001) Randomized phase III trial of paclitaxel plus carbonplatin versus vinorelbine plus cisplatin in the treatment of patients with advanced non-small-cell lung cancer: a Southwest Oncology Group trial. *Journal of Clinical Oncology* **19**: 3210–3218.

Klastersky J, Sculier JP, Dabouis G et al. (1990) A randomized trial of two platinum combinations in patients with advanced non-small cell lung cancer: a preliminary report. European Organization for the Research and Treatment of Cancer – Lung Cancer Working Party. *Seminars in Oncology* **17**(1 Suppl 2): 20–24.

Kosmidis P, Bacoyiannis C, Mylonakis N et al. (2000) A randomized phase III trial of paclitaxel plus carboplatin versus paclitaxel plus gemcitabine in advanced non small cell lung cancer (NSCLC) A preliminary analysis. *Proceedings of the American Society of Clinical Oncology* **20**: abstract 1908.

Langer C, Adak S, Thor A et al. (2001) Phase II Eastern Cooperative Oncology Group (ECOG) pilot study of paclitaxel (P), carboplatin (C), and trastuzumab (T) in HER-2/*neu* (+) advanced non-small cell lung cancer (NSCLC): Early analysis of E2598. *Proceedings of the American Society of Clinical Oncology* **20**: abstract 1257.

Lees M, Aristides M, Maniandakis N et al. (2002) Economic evaluation of gemcitabine alone and in combination with cisplatin in the treatment of Non-small Cell Lung Cancer. *Pharmacoeconomics* **20**(5): 325–337.

Levi F, Lucchini F, LaVecchia C et al. (1999) Trends in mortality from cancer in the European Union, 1955–94. *The Lancet* **354**: 742–743.

Macha HN, Gatzemeier U, Betticher DC et al. (1998) Randomized multicenter trial comparing paclitaxel (tax)/carboplatin (car) versus paclitaxel/cisplatin (cis) in advanced non-small cell lung cancer (NSCLC): Results of a planned interim analysis. *Proceedings of the American Society of Clinical Oncology* **17**(Meeting Abstract).

Manegold C, Drings P, von Pawel J et al. (1997) A randomized study of gemcitabine monotherapy versus etoposide/cisplatin in the treatment of locally advanced or metastatic non-small cell lung cancer. *Seminars in Oncology* **24**(3 suppl 8): S8-13–S8-17.

Martoni A, Guaraldi M, Piana E et al. (1998) Multicenter randomized clinical trial on high-dose epirubicin plus cis-platinum versus vinorelbine plus cis-platinum in advanced non small cell lung cancer. *Lung Cancer* **22**: 31–38.

Melo M, Barradas P, Costa A et al. (2002) Results of a randomised phase III trial comparing cisplatin (P)-based regimens in the treatment of locally advanced and metastatic non-small-cell lung cancer (NSCLC) mitomycin/cisplatin/vinblastine is no longer a therapeutic option. *Proceedings of the Annual Meeting of the American Society of Clinical Oncology* **21**: abstract 1205.

Non-small Cell Lung Cancer Collaborative Group (2001) Chemotherapy for non-small cell lung cancer (Cochrane Review). *The Cochrane Library*, Oxford Update Software.

Perng RP, Chen YM, Ming-Liu J et al. (1997) Gemcitabine versus the combination of cisplatin and etoposide in patients with inoperable non-small-cell lung cancer in a phase II randomized study. *Journal of Clinical Oncology* **15**: 2097–2102.

Ranson M, Davidson N, Nicolson M et al. (2000) Randomized trial of paclitaxel plus supportive care versus supportive care for patients with advanced non-small-cell lung cancer. *Journal of the National Cancer Institute* **92**: 1074–1080.

Rodriguez J, Pawel J, Pluzanska A et al. (2001) A multicenter, randomized phase III study of docetaxel + cisplatin (DC) and docetaxel + carboplatin (DCB) vs. vinorelbine + cisplatin (VC) in chemotherapy-naive patients with advanced and metastatic non-small cell lung cancer. *Proceedings of the American Society of Clinical Oncology* **20**: abstract 1252.

Rosso R, Ardizzoni A, Salvari F et al. (1988) Etoposide v etoposide and cisplatin in the treatment of advanced non-small cell lung cancer: a FONICAP randomized study. *Seminars in Oncology* **15**(6 suppl 7): 49–51.

Roszkowski K, Pluzanska A, Krzakowski M et al. (2000) A multicenter, randomized, phase III study of docetaxel plus best supportive care versus best supportive care in chemotherapy-naive patients with metastatic or non-resectable localized non-small cell lung cancer (NSCLC) *Lung Cancer* **27**: 145–157.

Sandler AB, Nemunaitis J, Denham C et al. (2000) Phase III trial of gemcitabine plus cisplatin versus cisplatin alone in patients with locally advanced or metastatic non-small-cell lung cancer. *Journal of Clinical Oncology* **18**: 122–130.

Scagliotti GV, De Marinis F, Rinaldi M et al. (2001) Phase III randomized trial comparing three platinum-based doublets in advanced non-small cell lung cancer. *Proceedings of the American Society of Clinical Oncology* **20**: abstract 1227.

Schiller JH, Harrington D, Belani CP et al. (2002) Comparison of four chemotherapy regimens for advanced non-small-cell lung cancer. *New England Journal of Medicine* **346**(2): 92–98.

Sederholm CJMF (2002) A phase III study in advanced non-small cell lung cancer (NSCLC) comparing gemcitabine (G) with gemcitabine in combination with carboplatin (C): Data from an ongoing study by the Swedish Lung Cancer Study Group (SLUSG). *Proceedings of the American Society of Clinical Oncology* **21**: abstract 1162.

Shepherd FA, Dancey J, Ramlan R et al. (2000) Prospective randomized trial of docetaxel versus best supportive care in patients with non-small-cell lung cancer previously treated with platinum-based chemotherapy. *Journal of Clinical Oncology* **18**: 2095–2103.

Smith IE, O'Brien ME, Talbot DC et al. (2001) Duration of chemotherapy in advanced non-small-cell lung cancer: a randomized trial of three versus six courses of mitomycin, vinblastine, and cisplatin. *Journal of Clinical Oncology* **19**: 1336–1343.

Socinski MA, Schell MJ, Peterman A et al. (2002) Phase III trial comparing a defined duration of therapy versus continuous therapy followed by second-line therapy in advanced-stage IIIB/IV NSCLC. *Journal of Clinical Oncology* **20**(5): 1335–1345.

Splinter TA, Sahmoud T, Festen J et al. (1996) Two schedules of teniposide with or without cisplatin in advanced non-small-cell lung cancer: a randomized study of the European Organization for Research and Treatment of Cancer Lung Cancer Cooperative Group. *Journal of Clinical Oncology* **14**: 127–134.

Takeda, K, N. Yamamoto, Negoro S et al. (2000) Randomized phase II study of docetaxel (DOC) plus cisplatin (CDDP) versus DOC plus irinotecan in advanced non-small-cell lung cancer (NSCLC); A West Japan Thoracic Oncology Group (WJTOG) Study. *Proceedings of the American Society of Clinical Oncology* **19**: abstract 1944.

Talbot D, White S, Jones P et al. (2000) Phase II Study of exatecan mesylate (DX-8951f) in advanced NSCLC. *Proceedings of the American Society of Clinical Oncology* **19**: abstract 2166.

ten Bokkel Huinink WW, Bergman B, Chemaissani A et al. (1999) Single-agent gemcitabine: an active and better tolerated alternative to standard cisplatin-based chemotherapy in locally advanced or metastatic non-small cell lung cancer. *Lung Cancer* **26**: 85–94.

Thompson DS, Hainsworth JD, Burris III HA et al. (2001) Prospective randomized study of four third generation chemotherapy regimens in patients (pts) with advanced non-small cell lung cancer: a Minnie Pearl Cancer Research Network Trial. *Proceedings of the American Society of Clinical Oncology* **20**: abstract 1253.

Thompson WJ, Piazza GA, Li H et al. (2000) Exisulind induction of apoptosis involves guanosine 3′,5′-cyclic monophosphate phosphodiesterase inhibition, protein kinase G activation, and attenuated beta-catenin. *Cancer Research* **60**: 3338–3342.

Treat J, Huang C, Damjanou N et al. (2001) Phase II monotherapy trial of ZD0473 as second-line therapy in non-small cell lung cancer. *Proceedings of the American Society of Clinical Oncology* **20**: abstract 2808.

Van Meerbeeck J, Smit E, Lianes P et al. (2001) A EORTC Randomized phase III trial of three chemotherapy regimens in advanced non-small cell lung cancer (NSCLC). *Proceedings of the American Society of Clinical Oncology* **20**: abstract 1228.

Veeder MH, Jett JR, Su JQ et al. (1992) A phase III trial of mitomycin C alone versus mitomycin C, vinblastine, and cisplatin for metastatic squamous cell lung carcinoma. *Cancer* **70**: 2281–2287.

Wozniak AJ, Crowley JJ, Balcerzak SP et al. (1998) Randomized trial comparing cisplatin with cisplatin plus vinorelbine in the treatment of advanced non-small-cell lung cancer: a Southwest Oncology Group study. *Journal of Clinical Oncology* **16**: 2459–2465.

Yuen A, Advani R, Fisher G et al. (2000) A phase I/II trial of ISIS 3521, an antisense inhibitor of protein kinase C alpha, combined with carboplatin and paclitaxel in patients with non-small cell lung cancer. *Proceedings of the American Society of Clinical Oncology* **19**: abstract 1802.

PART 4

Clinical trials and novel therapies

Generating new medical evidence for management: an overview of clinical trials in progress

Jeremy PC Steele and Robin M Rudd

Cure rates for lung cancer remain low. For non-small cell lung cancer (NSCLC) patients, cure can be achieved with radical surgery or radiotherapy; chemotherapy has not yet contributed significantly to the number of patients surviving. Chemotherapy can produce remissions in most patients with small cell lung cancer (SCLC), but ultimately only a small percentage are cured. In recent years, new drugs and new ways of delivering radiotherapy have led to optimism in the search for better results. Only well-organised clinical trials can establish the role of new therapies.

Clinical trials in lung cancer have several possible endpoints: overall survival, progression-free survival, response rate and quality of life. In most phase III trials – including the majority of those discussed here – all four endpoints are examined. It is our view that all trials should include evaluation of quality of life.

Most trials are performed according to phase II or III designs. In the UK, trials take place within single institutions or on a multicentre basis organised by groups such as the London Lung Cancer Group funded by the Cancer Research UK and the Medical Research Council (MRC). In mainland Europe, trials are conducted locally, nationally and internationally under the direction of groups such as the European Organisation for Research and Treatment of Cancer (EORTC). In North America, the US and Canadian National Cancer Institutes coordinate and fund many trials. Other well-known groups in the USA are the Southwest Oncology Group (SWOG), the Eastern Collaborative Oncology Group (ECOG) and the Cancer and Leukemia Group B (CALGB). Multicentre trials have the advantage of centralised randomisation and data analysis, and have the ability to recruit the large numbers of patients required for phase III studies.

This chapter describes some of the significant trials recruiting lung cancer patients in Europe and North America. The trials chosen are included because they are asking important questions. In each case the trial is put in the context of the existing evidence base and the specific question being asked is highlighted. Possible difficulties with accrual, where present, are discussed. Trials in NSCLC are described first, followed by SCLC.

Trials in non-small cell lung cancer

The standard treatment for medically fit patients with early stage NSCLC (stages I and II) is radical surgery with lobectomy or pneumonectomy. Radical thoracic radiotherapy can produce long-term cures in patients unsuitable for surgery. Stage IIIA NSCLC is resectable in some cases, but most patients will relapse and for patients with unresectable disease (stages IIIB and IV) the aim of treatment is symptom relief and prolongation of life (Non-small Cell Lung Cancer Collaborative Group 1995). Thus there is an ongoing need to evaluate new ways of treating patients with this common cancer.

What is the role of preoperative chemotherapy for patients with operable (i.e. stages I–IIIA) NSCLC?

NSCLC is responsive to chemotherapy, so preoperative chemotherapy may shrink the tumour and make subsequent surgery easier and safer. Theoretically, there may be a survival benefit by elimination of micrometastases.

Existing data have not made a clear argument for this approach: Roth et al. (1994) reported a benefit for preoperative chemotherapy, although the survival in the control arm (i.e. surgery only) appeared to be inferior to normal expectations. Rosell et al. (1994) described a similar result for patients treated with preoperative chemotherapy, although there was an excess of poor-prognosis features in the control arm. Depierre et al. (1999) reported a larger randomised trial in abstract form. Again the results were equivocal. Most investigators conclude that further trials are warranted.

MRC phase III randomised trial LU22 (UK)

Patients with resectable NSCLC are randomised to immediate surgery *or* to three cycles of preoperative cisplatin-based chemotherapy followed by surgery. Of the projected 450 patients, 180 have been randomised.

Intergroup phase III randomised trial 9900 (USA)

Patients with resectable NSCLC are randomised to immediate surgery *or* paclitaxel and carboplatin chemotherapy for up to three cycles, followed by surgery. Target accrual is 600 patients.

What is the role of postoperative chemotherapy and radiotherapy in NSCLC?

Adjuvant chemotherapy is effective in breast and colon cancer but its value in NSCLC is unclear. The theoretical advantages are better long-term survival rates by elimination of micrometastases and improved local control. Postoperative radiotherapy may also be beneficial, but current data do not support its use. A recent meta-analysis suggested that radiotherapy might be detrimental (PORT Meta-analysis

Trialists Group 1998). Trials attempting to answer these questions include the following.

Adjuvant Lung Project phase III trial (Italy + EORTC))

Patients with resected stages I–IIIA NSCLC were randomised to MVP (methotrexate–vinblastine–cisplatin) chemotherapy *or* no chemotherapy. Radiotherapy was given in either arm according to the physician's discretion. This trial closed in 2000 and will report in 2002.

International Adjuvant Lung Trial (Europe)

Patients with operable (stages I–IIIA) NSCLC are randomised to cisplatin-based chemotherapy *or* no chemotherapy after successful resection. Radiotherapy can be given to patients on either trial arm according to institutional guidelines. Accrual will be complete in 2003.

ANITA Studies (Europe)

Patients with operable NSCLC are randomised to chemotherapy *or* no chemotherapy after complete resection. In ANITA 1, chemotherapy is vinorelbine and cisplatin; in ANITA 2, it is single-agent vinorelbine. Radiotherapy is optional for patients with N2 disease. ANITA 1 has recently closed to recruitment.

National Cancer Institute of Canada phase III trial BR10 (North America)

Patients with resected T2N0 or T1–2N1 NSCLC were randomised to chemotherapy (vinorelbine and cisplatin for four cycles) *or* no further treatment. This trial closed in 2000 with 600 patients randomised.

CALGB phase III trial 9633 (USA)

Patients with stage IB NSCLC are randomised to paclitaxel and carboplatin chemotherapy *or* no further treatment. Target accrual is 500 patients.

What is the best treatment for inoperable stage IIIA NSCLC?

Patients with inoperable NSCLC are offered radical thoracic radiotherapy with curative intent, although there are few long-term survivors. There is therefore interest in adding chemotherapy for these patients to improve outcomes. Curran et al. (2000) showed that chemoradiotherapy given sequentially or synchronously was more effective than radiotherapy alone (median survival 13.7 months vs 11.4 months; 1-year survival rate 59% vs 46%).

Unresectable stage IIIA NSCLC: a comparison of standard radiotherapy with chemotherapy followed by radiotherapy (MRC LU20, UK)

Patients with untreated, unresectable stage IIIA NSCLC were randomised to receive standard thoracic radiotherapy *or* combination chemotherapy followed by radiotherapy or, if feasible, surgery. The target accrual was 350 patients over 3 years but the trial closed because of poor recruitment with 48 patients randomised.

As with many trials in which the treatments in the two arms are substantially different, this trial closed as a result of slow accrual. Also, patients with unresectable stage IIIA disease are a small proportion of NSCLC in the UK where most patients present with stage IIIB or IV disease.

Is surgery or radiotherapy better as definitive treatment for patients with resectable stage IIIA NSCLC responding to initial chemotherapy?

For patients with resectable stage IIIA NSCLC, surgery may offer a greater chance of cure than radiotherapy (Ginsberg et al. 1997). Retrospective data suggest superior survival rates for patients receiving surgery but this may be the result of patient selection. The EORTC are examining this issue in a randomised trial:

Chemotherapy followed by radiotherapy or surgery in stage IIIA NSCLC (EORTC 08941, Europe)

Patients with stage IIIA NSCLC receive three courses of platinum-based chemotherapy. Patients achieving complete or partial remission are randomised to surgery *or* radiotherapy (60 62.5 Gy). Postoperative radiotherapy is given to surgical patients if resection margins or nodes are positive for tumour. The target accrual is 800 patients in order to randomise 400 patients.

What is the benefit of chemotherapy with CHART for patients with stage III NSCLC?

Continuous hyperfractionated accelerated radiotherapy (CHART) is radiotherapy given more than once daily. Protocols have examined two or three times daily fractionation. Hyperfractionation theoretically produces improved tumour control as suggested by radiobiological models of tumour cell repopulation. The additional advantage is that the duration of the treatment period is shortened. Logistically, CHART places additional demands on radiotherapy departments and patients are required to remain in the hospital for the whole day. Despite the significant financial and organisational issues, there is interest in CHART in Europe and North America, because the original Mount Vernon trial showed improved overall survival and local control with acceptable toxicity (Saunders et al. 1997). Two ongoing trials are described.

Chemotherapy followed by standard or hyperfractionated radiotherapy for
unresectable stage IIIA or IIIB NSCLC (ECOG 2597, USA)

Patents with unresectable stage IIIA or IIIB NSCLC are treated with two cycles of paclitaxel and carboplatin chemotherapy. Responding patients and those with stable disease are randomised to standard *or* hyperfractionated (three fractions daily) radiotherapy. Target accrual is 300 patients over 3 years.

Phase II trial of CHART after chemotherapy (Mount Vernon, UK)

Patients with unresectable stage IIIA/IIIB NSCLC receive four cycles of cisplatin and paclitaxel followed by CHART.

What is the overall role of cisplatin-based chemotherapy in NSCLC and what are the quality-of-life benefits?

The London Lung Cancer Group (LLCG) 'Big Lung Trial' explored the role of cisplatin-based based chemotherapy in all stages of NSCLC. This large project allowed investigators to randomise between the addition of chemotherapy and no further therapy for any patient with NSCLC for whom the value of chemotherapy is perceived to be uncertain or marginal.

Trial of cisplatin-based chemotherapy in NSCLC (LLCG BLT, Europe)

This is a randomised trial to determine the value of cisplatin-based chemotherapy in NSCLC of any stage. Patients had received surgery or radiotherapy or both, or had advanced disease unsuitable for radical local therapy. In all settings, the randomisation was between chemotherapy and no chemotherapy. Chemotherapy can be MIC (mitomycin, ifosfamide and cisplatin), MVP, cisplatin/vindesine (CV) or cisplatin/vinorelbine (NP). Endpoints were: survival, progression-free survival, quality of life and health economics. The trial closed in November 2001 with over 1000 patients randomised. Early results should be available in 2002.

Are newer drugs better and less toxic than existing agents?

Several new chemotherapy drugs have emerged in the last few years, some of which have shown useful activity in common solid tumours in adults. The most important of these are docetaxel, gemcitabine, irinotecan, paclitaxel, topotecan and vinorelbine. These newer agents have the advantage of being less toxic than older drugs. The significant drawback is that the newer agents are several times the cost of the drugs that they may supersede, but have been associated with less hospitalisation. Trials are ongoing that aim to determine the exact role of these newer drugs.

Phase III trial comparing gemcitabine/carboplatin with mitomycin/ifosfamide/cisplatin in stage IIIB or IV NSCLC (London Lung Cancer Group Study 11, UK)

Patients received chemotherapy with gemcitabine and carboplatin *or* MIC. Endpoints were quality of life and survival. This trial completed 8 months earlier than anticipated with over 300 patients randomised. Preliminary results show improved survival, less toxicity and better quality of life for the gemcitabine and carboplatin arm (Rudd et al. 2002).

Trials in small cell lung cancer

The chemosensitivity of SCLC is well known and most patients – regardless of initial disease bulk – can be expected to achieve a remission. However, only a small percentage (approximately 5%) of individuals are cured – relapse after a period of months or years is the norm. Clinical trials are aiming to prolong the progression-free period and increase the number of cures. The following are important questions that need to be answered.

What is the role of higher intensity treatment in patients with limited-disease SCLC?

There has been interest in dose-intensified treatment for patients with SCLC for some years, but results have not been clear-cut (Elias 1998). A platinum-containing protocol is the current gold standard and higher-dose or higher-intensity therapy should be used only in clinical trials. Most interest is centred on higher-intensity chemotherapy rather than classic high-dose therapy. Typically, growth factors are employed to allow chemotherapy cycles to be given 2-weekly rather than 3-weekly.

Phase II study of intensive chemotherapy with peripheral blood progenitor cell support in SCLC (EU 98072, Europe)

Patients with good prognosis SCLC are treated with four 14-day cycles of ifosfamide, carboplatin and etoposide; granulocyte colony-stimulating factor (G-CSF) is given until blood counts recover. Peripheral blood progenitor cells are reinfused after cycles 2 and 3. Patients achieving complete remission will receive prophylactic cranial radiotherapy.

Randomised clinical trial of 'V-ICE' chemotherapy versus standard treatment in SCLC (MRC LU21 trial, UK)

Patients with limited-disease SCLC or good-prognosis extensive SCLC receive six courses of intensive V-ICE chemotherapy (ifosfamide 5 g/m^2, carboplatin 300 mg/m^2, etoposide 120 mg/m^2 on day 1 and vincristine 1 mg/m^2 on day 14, repeated every 28 days) *or* standard chemotherapy (ACE [doxorubicin, cyclophosphamide and etoposide] or PE [cisplatin and etoposide]) for six courses. This trial will close in December 2001 with 400 patients recruited.

When should radiotherapy be administered in limited-disease SCLC?

Data have suggested that thoracic radiotherapy for patients with limited-disease SCLC is more beneficial if administered synchronously (Murray et al. 1993), although acute toxicity is greater. The trial described below will clarify the issue:

Phase III trial to examine the timing of radiotherapy in limited-disease SCLC (London Lung Cancer Group Study 8, UK)

Patients with limited-disease SCLC were treated with CAV/PE (cyclophosphamide, doxorubicin and vincristine alternating with cisplatin and etoposide) chemotherapy and prophylactic cranial radiotherapy, and were randomised to 40 Gy of thoracic radiotherapy given after the first cycle of PE *or* after the third cycle of PE. This trial will close in December 2001 with over 300 patients randomised.

What is the benefit of newer chemotherapy agents?

Newer agents such as docetaxel, gemcitabine, irinotecan, paclitaxel, topotecan and vinorelbine have demonstrated activity in SCLC and are being tested in randomised trials. All of these agents appear to have useful single-agent activity in SCLC, but are considerably more expensive than existing drugs.

Phase III study of etoposide and cisplatin with or without paclitaxel in extensive-disease SCLC (NCI and CALGB 9732, USA)

Patients with extensive-disease SCLC are randomised to six 3-weekly cycles of cisplatin and etoposide *or* cisplatin, etoposide and paclitaxel. Target accrual is 670 patients over 16 months.

Gemcitabine and carboplatin compared with cisplatin and etoposide in extensive disease and poor-prognosis limited disease SCLC patients (London Lung Cancer Group Study 10, UK)

Patients with SCLC (extensive disease or limited disease with poor-prognosis factors) were randomised to six cycles of gemcitabine and carboplatin *or* six cycles of cisplatin and etoposide. Endpoints were response rate, quality of life and survival. This trial closed in September 2001 and initial results show that the two protocols produced similar survival results but with less toxicity for the gemcitabine/carboplatin combination (James et al. 2002).

Should second-line therapy for patients with SCLC be routine?

Second-line treatment for patients with SCLC may produce significant symptomatic benefit for selected patients. One approach is to re-treat the patient with a platinum-based combination, although some centres are investigating the role of newer, non-cross-resistant agents.

Phase II trial of irinotecan, cisplatin and mitomycin in relapsed SCLC (St Bartholomew's Hospital, London)

Patients with recurrent SCLC are treated with irinotecan 70 mg/m^2 and cisplatin 40 mg/m^2 2-weekly and mitomycin C 6 mg/m^2 4-weekly for up to six cycles according to response. Target accrual is 24 patients.

Phase II trial of topotecan and paclitaxel in relapsed SCLC (NCI, USA)

Patients with recurrent SCLC are treated with paclitaxel and topotecan in cohorts, with escalating doses of topotecan for a maximum of six courses.

Are new treatment modalities of value?

As standard cytotoxic treatments have such low cure rates, SCLC and NSCLC are ideal diseases in which to assess experimental drugs. Novel approaches such as anti-angiogenesis, monoclonal antibody targeting and gene therapy are being evaluated. In most countries gene therapy protocols are monitored by government agencies. Examples of novel agents that are in phase II or III trials are shown in Table 7.1.

Table 7.1 Novel agents in phase II or III trials

Molecular/cellular target	Examples of drugs
Epidermal growth factor receptor	Iressa (ZD1839), C225: Herceptin (trastuzumab)
Ras oncogene	Anti-ras anti-sense oligonucleotides
Farnesyl transferase	Farnesyl transferase inhibitors (FTIs)
Vascular endothelial growth factor receptor (VEGF)	VEGF receptor antibodies
Angiogenesis and cytokine networks	Thalidomide

Conclusions

There are many lung cancer clinical trials in progress in North America, Europe and other countries. If recruitment to trials continues, it is possible that many of the important questions regarding the best management of NSCLC and SCLC with surgery, chemotherapy and radiotherapy will be answered in the next few years. New modalities of therapy offer promise, but most are at an early stage of development. It is our view that clinical trials should receive maximal support from governments, healthcare systems and physicians. As many patients as possible should have the opportunity to be treated within a clinical trial.

References

Curran WJ, Scott C, Langer C et al. (2000) Phase III comparison of sequential vs concurrent chemoradiation for patients with unresected stage III non-small cell lung cancer (NSCLC): initial report of radiation oncology group (RTOG) 9410. *Proceedings of the American Society of Clinical Oncology* **19**: abstract 1891.

Depierre A, Milleron B, Moro SD et al. (1999) Phase III Trial of neo-adjuvant chemotherapy in respectable stage I (except T1N1), II, IIIa non-small cell lung cancer (NSCLC): the French experience. *Proceedings of the American Society of Clinical Oncology* **18**: abstract 1792.

Elias A (1998) Dose-intensive therapy in small cell lung cancer. *Chest* **113**(1 suppl), 101S–106S.

Ginsberg RJ, Vokes EE, Raben A (1997) Non-small cell lung cancer. In: DeVita VT, Hellman S, Rosenberg SA (eds), *Cancer, Principles and Practice of Oncology*, 5th edn. Philadelphia: Lippincott-Raven, pp. 858–911.

James LE, Rudd R, Gower NH et al. (2002) A phase III randomised comparison of gemcitabine/carboplatin (GC) with cisplatin/etoposide (PE) in patients with poor prognosis small cell lung cancer (SCLC). *Proceedings of the American Society of Clinical Oncology* **21**: abstract 1170.

Murray N, Coy P, Pater JL et al. (1993) Importance of timing for thoracic irradiation in the combined modality treatment of limited-stage small-cell lung cancer. The National Cancer Institute of Canada Clinical Trials Group. *Journal of Clinical Oncology* **11**: 336–344.

Non-small Cell Lung Cancer Collaborative Group (1995) Chemotherapy in non-small cell lung cancer: a meta-analysis using updated data on individual patients from 52 randomised clinical trials. *British Medical Journal* **311**: 899–909.

PORT Meta-analysis Trialists Group (1998) Postoperative radiotherapy in non-small-cell lung cancer: systematic review and meta-analysis of individual patient data from nine randomised trials. *The Lancet* **352**: 257–263.

Roth JA, Fossella F, Komaki R et al. (1994) A randomized trial comparing perioperative chemotherapy and surgery with surgery alone in resectable stage IIIA non-small-cell lung cancer. *Journal of the National Cancer Institute* **86**: 673–680.

Rosell R, Gomez-Codina J, Camps C et al. (1994) A randomized trial comparing preoperative chemotherapy plus surgery with surgery alone in patients with non-small-cell lung cancer. *New England Journal of Medicine* **330**: 153–158.

Rudd R, Gower N, James L et al. (2002) Phase III randomised comparison of gemcitabine and carboplatin with mitomycin, ifosfamide and cisplatin in advanced NSCLC. *Proceedings of the American Society of Clinical Oncology* **21**: abstract 1164.

Saunders M, Dische S, Barrett A et al. (1997) Continuous hyperfractionated accelerated radiotherapy (CHART) versus conventional radiotherapy in non-small-cell lung cancer: a randomised multicentre trial. *The Lancet* **350**: 161–165.

Chapter 8

Biological approaches to the management of lung cancer: the theoretical basis and clinical significance of novel therapies targeting the epidermal growth factor receptor

Malcolm Ranson, G Jayson and N Thatcher

Although non-specific cytotoxic drugs have brought significant advances in the treatment of cancer, we may be approaching a therapeutic plateau for non-selective cytotoxic drugs in the treatment of some common epithelial tumours, including non-small cell lung cancer (NSCLC).

The recent development of highly selective, target-based cancer therapeutics has resulted from a greater understanding of tumour biology. Agents that target critical components of cell signalling, angiogenesis, cell cycle control and metastasis are now under clinical evaluation and some of these agents have begun to show significant promise.

The challenge in developing these agents is to understand that these drugs will require a re-evaluation of the traditional concepts of anti-cancer drug development that have previously been applied to cytotoxic drugs.

Dose–toxicity relationships may be less steep and therapeutic windows wider than for cytotoxic drugs, rendering less useful traditional endpoints in phase I trials such as maximum tolerable dose (MTD). More relevant endpoints in early clinical trials may be the identification of biologically active dose ranges, or the definition of an optimal biological dose. The primary endpoint in phase II trials of cytotoxic anti-cancer drugs is the proportion of patients showing tumour regression ('response rate'). This endpoint is likely to be less relevant for novel target-specific agents. Endpoints that reflect 'tumour control', such as time to tumour progression, survival, quality of life and improvement in disease-related symptoms, are likely to be more relevant. However, accurate determination of these endpoints requires larger randomised trials with a comparator arm. In determining which agents to prioritise for phase III evaluation, well-designed early clinical trials are paramount. Techniques that allow early readout of biological effect using direct or surrogate measurements are now available (e.g. biopsy assessment of drug target inhibition, positron emission tomography and dynamic magnetic resonance). These techniques will need to be validated as being reliable predictors of altered tumour growth, tumour regression and clinical outcome. Thus, rational development of these novel compounds will require investment in translational research.

A wide range of new agents that have potential in lung cancer treatment is in development, but the clinical utility of some of the proposed targets has yet to be validated in a clinical setting. Among the most promising of new agents in NSCLC are inhibitors of the epidermal growth factor receptor (EGFR) system and these new agents will be the focus of this overview.

Epidermal growth factor receptor

The epidermal growth factor family is composed of four closely related receptors (EGFR, HER2, HER3, HER4) (Mendelsohn and Baselga 2000; Woodburn 1999). The most widely expressed of the EGFR family members in human cancer is EGFR. Multiple ligands for EGFR have been identified including EGF, tumour growth factor α (TGFα), amphiregulin, epiregulin and heparin-binding EGF. The EGFR can be divided into three structural domains: an extracellular domain, a transmembrane region and an intracellular domain (Figure 8.1). The extracellular domain of the EGF family of receptors contains two cysteine-rich regions and binds to EGF-related growth factors. The intracellular portion contains a tyrosine kinase domain and docking sites for additional kinase substrates. Ligand binding to the extracellular domain of the receptor triggers receptor dimerisation, and activates intracellular tyrosine kinase domains on each to transphosphorylate tyrosine residues on the other EGFR molecule. These activated domains act as binding sites for adapter proteins triggering a signal transduction cascade (Figure 8.2).

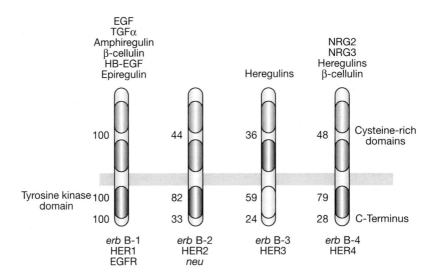

Figure 8.1 The epidermal growth factor receptor (ErbB) family and their ligands.

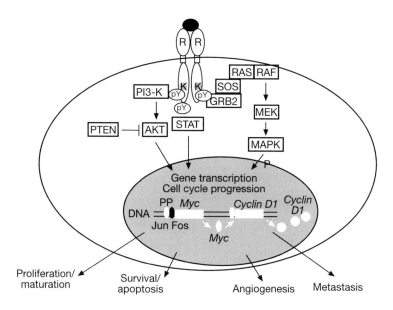

Figure 8.2 Epidermal growth factor receptor (EGFR) signal transduction in tumour cells.

Multiple EGFR-linked intracellular signalling pathways have been described and are reviewed elsewhere (Enis et al. 1991; Moghal and Sternberg 1999). In epithelial tissues and tumours, the EGFR seems to be a crucial element in integrating information from multiple receptor pathways via receptor cross-talk or transactivation, e.g. transactivation resulting in EGFR tyrosine phosphorylation can occur as part of cellular response to activation of G-protein-coupled receptors, radiation, oxidants and chemotherapeutic agents (Yamauchi et al. 1997; Hackel et al. 1999; Prenzel et al. 1999, 2000).

EGFR is widely expressed in human solid tumours (Salomon et al. 1995; Woodburn 1999) and there is considerable evidence that EGFR expression is linked to aberrant growth and cellular behaviour. Preclinical studies have demonstrated a link between elevated levels of EGFR expression and tumorigenesis (Velu 1990; Salomon et al. 1995). In addition, a number of EGFR mutations have been identified in human cancer, and these alterations result in altered expression of the extracellular ligand-binding domain of the receptor. The most common mutation is *EGFRvIII* and this receptor has a constitutive active tyrosine kinase domain. This mutant receptor is expressed in more than 50% of gliomas, as well as about 15% of cases of NSCLC (Ekstrand et al. 1994; Wikstrand et al. 1995, 1997; Chu et al. 1997; Voldborg et al. 1997; Olapade-Olaopa et al. 2000).

Many human epithelial tumours including NSCLC express elevated levels of EGFR and one or more of its ligands, suggesting that autocrine and paracrine loops occur commonly in human malignancy (Salomon et al. 1995; Fujino et al. 1996; Rusch et al. 1997; Fontanini et al. 1998). However, it is not clear if such loops are of crucial importance in the malignant phenotype. Nevertheless, in NSCLC, EGFR expression has been correlated with shorter overall survival (Volm et al. 1998), poor prognosis (Veale et al. 1993), a greater likelihood of metastases (Pravelic 1993) and increasing tumour stage (Fujino et al. 1996). The EGFR ligand amphiregulin has also been shown in multivariate analysis to correlate with reduced overall survival in NSCLC (Fontanini et al. 1998). Thus, it is probable that inhibiting the function of the EGFR may be therapeutically useful.

During solid tumour growth, the development of new vasculature occurs. EGF ligands and EGFR appear to contribute to this process. Both ligands and receptor have been shown to induce secondary angiogenesis in vivo in animal models (Schreiber et al. 1986). Multiple studies with EGFR inhibitors have also shown that inhibitors of EGFR are able to down-regulate angiogenesis by reducing expression of angiogenic factors such as VEGF (Schreiber et al. 1986; Viloria Petit et al. 1997; Perotte et al. 1999). Finally, both EGFR and its ligands have been shown to promote tumour cell mobility and invasion (reviewed in Woodburn 1999).

There is growing evidence to link EGFR expression with increased resistance to a number of anti-cancer drugs (Dickstein et al. 1993, 1995; Fischer-Colbrie et al. 1997). The combination of EGFR inhibition with cytotoxic drugs or with radiotherapy has been shown in animal tumour models to result in enhanced tumour control compared with these treatment modalities alone (Fan et al. 1993; Prewett et al. 1996; Mendelsohn and Fan 1997; Bruns et al. 1999; Ciardiello et al. 1999; Dent et al. 1999; Harari et al. 1999; Rao and Ethier 1999; Raben et al. 1999; Trumell et al. 1999; Milas et al. 2000; Wen et al. 2000a).

Multiple approaches have been used to search for anti-EGFR-selective drugs. Anti-EGFR-blocking monoclonal antibodies and fusion molecules containing EGFR ligands with potent toxins have been developed (Masui et al. 1989; Modjthedi et al. 1993; Arteaga et al. 1994; Schmidt and Wels 1996; Aboud-Pirak et al. 1998; Fan and Mendelsohn 1998). These biological approaches are targeted against the extracellular domain of the receptor. An alternative approach has been the development of agents that block the function of the receptor post-ligand binding. Multiple compounds of this type have been developed and a number of selective EGFR tyrosine kinase inhibitors have also been developed and tested clinically. The most extensively studied agents are C225 and ZD1839 and these are discussed further below.

C225 (cetuximab)

A series of murine monoclonal antibodies was produced in the 1980s (Sato et al. 1983), but the potential for development of human anti-mouse antibodies hindered their successful use in clinical trials. This problem has been overcome by the development of chimaeric and fully humanised monoclonal antibodies. The most extensively studied of these antibodies is C225 (cetuximab).

C225 is a chimaeric antibody which binds to the extracellular domain of the EGFR with greater affinity than the natural ligands, and results in decreased receptor activation and promotion of receptor internalisation (Sunada et al. 1986; Goldstein et al. 1995). The antibody C225 has been shown to inhibit a wide range of tumour cell lines in vitro and to have single-agent activity in animal models in tumours expressing EGFR (Masui et al. 1984; Rodeck et al. 1987; Goldstein et al. 1995; Aboud-Pirak et al. 1998). Preclinical studies in vitro and in vivo have shown that C225 enhances the anti-tumour effects of radiotherapy and chemotherapy treatments (Baselga et al. 1993; Ciardiello et al. 1999; Wen et al. 2000a). C225-induced blockade of the EGFR results in DNA-damaged cells undergoing cell cycle arrest and increased apoptosis. Agents such as C225 may well have significant potential to improve outcomes in lung cancer, particularly when used in conjunction with radiotherapy and chemotherapy.

As has been mentioned, the sensitivity of tumours to chemotherapeutic drugs can be influenced by EGFR blockade. Monoclonal antibodies such as C225 enhance the cytotoxic activity of cisplatin, paclitaxel, gemcitabine, topotecan, vinorelbine and doxorubicin in preclinical models (Prewett et al. 1996; Ciardiello et al. 1999; Huang et al. 1999).

C225 is administered intravenously and has been evaluated in early clinical trials in over 600 patients. It is generally well tolerated. The most common toxicity is of an acneiform skin rash, which typically appears during the first few weeks of treatment and is reversible on withdrawal of treatment. Occasional instances of allergic reaction have been reported with C225 and thus, initially, a test dose of antibody is frequently deployed. Most of the studies performed to date have been dose-ranging phase I/II studies to define the pharmacokinetic and toxicity profile of the antibody. The approach in the phase II and III trials to date has been to focus on patients known to have EGFR expression or overexpression. This is based on preclinical data and the expectation that C225 will have activity primarily in receptor-positive patients. The studies to date show that C225 has non-linear pharmacokinetics and that a dosing schedule of 400 mg/m^2 loading and 250 mg/m^2 weekly maintenance is likely to be well tolerated by patients and to achieve relatively sustained levels of EGFR blockade. However, large randomised phase III trials have not evaluated whether less frequent dosing strategies may yield equivalent clinical outcomes. Phase II trials have focused on patients with advanced-stage squamous cell head and neck cancer, NSCLC, colorectal cancer and pancreatic cancer. Trials in advanced NSCLC are under way in combination with carboplatin/paclitaxel and carboplatin/gemcitabine.

ZD1839 (iressa)

ZD1839 is an orally active quinazoline EGFR tyrosine kinase inhibitor, which is now in phase III trials in NSCLC and also under investigation in a wide range of other tumour types. ZD1839 monotherapy is in phase I trials and preliminary phase II experience in relapsed advanced NSCLC. ZD1839 has been studied in four separate phase I trials in patients with advanced refractory tumours. After oral administration, ZD1839 is well absorbed and plasma levels of the drug decline biphasically with the terminal half-life of 12–50 hours (Kelly et al. 2000), allowing drug levels to be easily maintained by once-daily tablet administration.

Preliminary data from these phase I studies are available. A total of 252 patients were recruited to the four trials, including 100 patients with advanced, relapsed NSCLC. Most patients were heavily pre-treated. ZD1839 appeared to be well tolerated at doses up to 70 mg/day. The most frequent adverse effects were of diarrhoea, acne-like skin rash and mild nausea. Patients were monitored for ophthalmic changes by slit-lamp examinations, but there was no evidence of consistent or drug-related ophthalmic effects. Occasional instances of reversible transaminase increases have been noted in some patients. Grade 3 and 4 adverse drug effects were uncommon below 600 mg/day and dose-limiting toxicity comprised diarrhoea in the dose-escalation trials. Skin rash and diarrhoea are reversible on drug withdrawal or on dose reduction.

Evidence of anti-tumour activity in advanced refractory NSCLC has been reported from the phase I trials, with anti-tumour activity seen across a wide range of doses (Baselga et al. 2000; Ferry et al. 2000; Nakagawa et al. 2000; Negoro et al. 2001). A single optimal biological dose could not be defined from the phase I studies and thus two dose levels (250 mg and 500 mg/day) were selected for further evaluation in advanced NSCLC. A dose of 250 mg/day achieved plasma levels that would be expected to result in EGFR blockade based on the pre-clinical data for ZD1839, and 500 mg/day, although associated with a greater incidence of dose interruptions, was tolerable by most patients on long-term administration.

Early results of a large phase II trial in patients with advanced NSCLC who had failed one or two prior chemotherapy regimens has recently been reported in abstract form (Baselga et al. 2001). In this study patients who had failed one or two prior regimens for advanced NSCLC (including a platinum-containing regimen) were randomised in a double-masked multicentre trial to ZD1839 either 250 mg/day or 500 mg/day. A total of 210 patients was randomised and 208 patients were evaluable for response at the time of reporting. The overall tumour response was 18.7% (95%CI 13.7–24.7), the tumour response rate being very similar for second-line and third-line treatment. Median progression free survival was 84 days and 34% of patients were still progression-free at 4 months. Meaningful survival data were not available because the follow-up on this trial at the time of reporting was short and the median survival had not been reached. Disease-related symptoms were assessed by the FACT-LCS scale, and this showed that 39% of patients showed an overall improvement in disease-related symptoms. An important finding from this trial was that there was no difference in the tumour efficacy endpoints between 250 and 500 mg/day. Both dose levels were well tolerated but the incidence of treatment-limiting toxicity was significantly lower with 250 mg/day than with 500 mg/day.

These results compare relatively favourably with the results obtained from multicentre trials of docetaxel, the only agent so far to have shown consistent activity as a second-line treatment of advanced NSCLC. These early data provide a strong rationale for the further study of ZD1839 in patients with NSCLC, both as monotherapy and in combination. Information on the relationship of EGFR expression to clinical outcome is awaited. Preclinical data showing that EGFR blockade enhances the efficacy of cytotoxic agents have been discussed above and, given the single-agent activity of ZD1839 combinations of ZD1839 with cytotoxic drug regimens, they are of considerable interest.

Combination therapy with ZD1839 in NSCLC

ZD1839 is currently being evaluated in combination with a range of cytotoxic agents. Early results of a phase I trial of ZD1839 in combination with cisplatin/gemcitabine indicated that this combination had manageable and predictable toxicity, and in this phase I trial four of eight patients with advanced NSCLC achieved a partial response (Giaccone et al. 2001). The tolerability of ZD1839 has also been evaluated in phase I trial combined with carboplatin and paclitaxel. Results indicated that ZD1839 can be added to standard carboplatin/paclitaxel regimens without significantly increasing the overall toxicity (Miller et al. 2001).

ZD1839 in combination with either cisplatin/gemcitabine or carboplatin/paclitaxel is being investigated in two large multicentre randomised phase III trials in advanced NSCLC. Full results were presented at ESMO 2002.

In the clinical development of ZD1839, it is worth noting that patients have not been pre-selected based on tumour EGFR expression. It will be important to establish whether clinical benefit from ZD1839 either as monotherapy or in combination is related to pre-treatment EGFR expression. Given that EGFR signalling in tumours may be altered by the concurrent administration of cytotoxic therapy and the fact that multiple mutant receptors have been described, it will be important to see if a pre-treatment biopsy to determine EGFR status is of prognostic importance.

Conclusions

EGFR-targeted approaches to cancer treatment hold considerable promise. EGFR and its ligands play an important role in tumour growth and survival. The receptor system has been implicated in tumour development and progression. EGFR has an important influence on abnormal cellular proliferation, protection from apoptosis, angiogenesis and invasion, and metastasis. The combined results of studies to investigate the relationship between EGFR status in human cancers indicate a role in determining prognosis and responsiveness to existing modalities of treatment. The development of prognostic profiling of patients using data to relate treatment outcome to biological variables should help to define more rational therapeutic choices for patients in the future. It is anticipated that more information on the relationship between biological profiles and responsiveness to EGFR-targeted therapies will emerge from the ongoing clinical trials. Research is also attempting to identify potential mechanisms that may mediate resistance to EGFR-targeted therapies.

Clinical trials with multiple EGFR inhibitors are ongoing, using these agents as monotherapy as well as in combination with chemotherapy and radiotherapy. The focus of attention to date has been on the use of EGFR inhibitors in late-stage tumours and patients with metastatic disease. The tolerability and toxicity profile of these agents will undoubtedly facilitate their early investigation in early-stage disease and even in tumour prevention strategies in high-risk patients.

References

Aboud-Pirak E, Hurwitz E, Pirak ME et al. (1998) Efficacy of antibodies to epidermal growth factor receptor against KB carcinoma in vitro and in nude mice. *Journal of the National Cancer Institute* **80**: 1605–1611.

Arteaga CL, Hurd SD, Dugger TC et al. (1994) Epidermal growth factor receptors in human breast carcinoma cells: a potential selective target for transforming growth factor α-pseudomonas exotoxin 40 fusion protein. *Cancer Research* **54**: 4703–470.

Baselga J, Norton L, Masui H et al. (1993) Antitumour effects of doxorubicin in combination with anti-epidermal growth factor receptor monoclonal antibodies. *Journal of the National Cancer Institute* **85**: 1327–1333.

Baselga J, Herbst R, LoRusso P et al. (2000) Continuous administration of ZD1839 (Iressa) a novel oral epidermal growth factor receptor tyrosine kinase inhibitor in patients with five selected tumour types: evidence of activity and good tolerability. *Proceedings of the American Society of Clinical Oncology* **19**: 686 (abstract).

Baselga J, Yano S, Giaccone G et al. (2001) Initial results from a phase II trial of ZD1839 (Iressa) as second and third line monotherapy for patients with advanced non-small cell lung cancer. NCI-EORTC, Miami October (abstract).

Bruns CJ, Portera CA, Tsan RDJ et al. (1999) Regression of human pancreatic carcinoma growing orthotopically in athymic nude mice by blockade of epidermal growth factor receptor signalling in combination with gemcitabine. *Proceedings of the American Association for Cancer Research* **40**: 154 (abstract).

Chu CT, Everiss KD, Wikstrand CJ et al. (1997) Receptor dimerization is not a factor in the signalling activity of a transforming variant epidermal growth factor receptor (EGFRvIII). *Biochemical Journal* **324**: 855–861.

Ciardiello F, Bianco R, Damiano V et al. (1999) Antitumour activity of sequential treatment with topotecan and anti-epidermal growth factor receptor antibody C225. *Clinical Cancer Research* **5**: 909–916.

Ciardiello F, Caputo R, Bianco R et al. (2000) Antitumour effect and potentiation of cytotoxic drug activity in human cancer cells by ZD1839 (Iressa), an epidermal growth factor receptor selective tyrosine kinase inhibitor. *Clinical Cancer Research* **6**: 2053–2063.

Dent P, Reardon DB, Park JS et al. (1999) Radiation-induced release of transforming growth factor a activates the epidermal growth factor receptor and mitogen activated protein kinase pathway in carcinoma cells leading to increased proliferation and protection from radiation-induced cell death. *Molecular and Cell Biology* **10**: 2493–2506.

Dickstein BM, Valverius EM, Wosikowski K et al. (1993) Increased epidermal growth factor receptor in an oestrogen-responsive Adriamycin resistant MCF-7 cell line. *Journal of Cell Physiology* **157**: 110–118.

Dickstein BM, Wosikowski K, Bates SE (1995) Increased resistance to cytotoxic agents in ZR75B human breast cancer cells transfected with epidermal growth factor receptor. *Molecular and Cellular Endocrinology* **110**: 205–211.

Ekstrand AJ, Longo N, Hamid ML et al. (1994) Functional characterization of an EGF receptor with truncated extracellular domain expressed in glioblastomas with EGFR amplification. *Oncogene* **9**: 2313–2320.

Enis BW, Lippman ME, Dickson RB (1991) The EGF receptor system as a target for antitumour therapy. *Cancer Investigation* **9**: 553–562.

Fan Z, Baselga J, Masui H, Mendelsohn J (1993) Antitumour effect of anti-epidermal growth factor antibodies plus cisdiaminedichloroplatinum on well established A431 cell xenografts. *Cancer Research* **53**: 4637–4642.

Fan Z, Mendelsohn J (1998) Therapeutic application of anti growth factor receptor antibodies. *Current Opinions in Oncology* **10**: 67–73.

Ferry D, Hammond L, Ranson M et al. (2000) Intermittent oral Zd1839 (Iressa) a novel epidermal growth factor receptor tyrosine kinase inhibitor, shows evidence of good tolerability and activity: final results from a phase I study. *Proceedings of the American Society of Clinical Oncology* **19**: 5 (abstract)

Fischer-Colbrie J, Witt A, Heinzl H et al. (1997) EGFR and steroid receptors in ovarian carcinoma: comparison with prognostic parameters and outcome of patients. *Anticancer Research* **17**: 613–620.

Fontanini G, De Laurentis M, Vignati S (1998) Evaluation of epidermal growth factor related growth factors and receptors and of neoangiogenesis in completely resected stage I–IIIA non-small cell lung cancer: amphiregulin and microvessel count are independent prognostic indicators of survival. *Clinical Cancer Research* **4**: 241–249.

Fujino S, Enokibori T, Tezuka N et al. (1996) A comparison of epidermal growth factor receptor levels and other prognostic parameters in non-small cell lung cancer. *European Journal of Cancer* **32**: 2070–2074.

Giaconne G, Gonzales-Larriba JL, Smit EF et al. (2001) ZD1839 (Iressa) an orally active selective epidermal growth factor receptor tyrosine kinase inhibitor is well tolerated in combination with gemcitabine and cisplatin in patients with advanced solid tumours: preliminary tolerability, efficacy and pharmacokinetic studies. *European Journal of Cancer* **37**(suppl 6): 102 (abstract).

Goldstein NI, Prewett M, Zuklys K et al. (1995) Biological efficacy of a chimeric antibody to the epidermal growth factor receptor in a human xenograft model. *Clinical Cancer Research* **1**: 1311–1318.

Hackel PO, Zwick E, Prenzel N, Ulrich A (1999) Epidermal growth factor receptors: critical mediators of multiple receptor pathways. *Current Opinions in Cell Biology* **11**: 184–189.

Harari PM, Huang S, Li J (1999) Combining radiation with molecular blockade of the EGF receptor in cancer therapy. International Conference on Clinical Cancer Research. *Proceedings of the American Association of Cancer Research NCI-EORTC* **5**: 88 (abstract).

Huang SM, Bock JM, Harari PM et al. (1999) Epidermal growth factor receptor blockade with C225 modulates proliferation apoptosis and radiosensitivity in squamous cell carcinomas of the head and neck. *Cancer Research* **59**: 1935–1940.

Kelly HC, Ferry D, Hammond L et al. (2000) ZD1839 (Iressa) an oral EGFR-TKI: pharmacokinetics in a phase I study of patients with advanced cancer. *Proceedings of the American Association of Cancer Research* **41**: 3896 (abstract)

Masui H, Kawamoto T, Sato JD et al. (1984) Growth inhibition of human tumour cells in athymic mice by anti-epidermal growth factor receptor monoclonal antibodies. *Cancer Research* **44**: 1002–1007.

Masui H, Kamrath H, Apell G et al. (1989) Cytotoxicity against human tumour cells mediated by the conjugate of anti-epidermal growth factor receptor antibody to recombinant ricin A chain. *Cancer Research* **49**: 3482–3488

Mendelsohn J, Fan Z (1997) Epidermal growth factor receptor family and chemosensitisation. *Journal of the National Cancer Institute* **89**: 341–343.

Mendelson J, Baselga J (2000) The EGF receptor family as targets for cancer therapy. *Oncogene* **19**: 6550–6565.

Milas L, Mason K, Hunter N et al. (2000) In vivo enhancement of tumour radioresponse by C225 antiepidermal growth factor receptor antibody. *Clinical Cancer Research* **6**: 701–708.

Miller VA, Johnson D, Heelan RT et al. (2001) A pilot trial demonstrates the safety of ZD1839 (Iressa) an oral epidermal growth factor receptor tyrosine kinase inhibitor in combination with carboplatin and paclitaxel in previously untreated advanced non-small cell lung cancer. *Proceedings of the American Society of Clinical Oncology* **20**: 1301 (abstract).

Modjthedi H, Eccles S, Box G et al. (1993) Immunotherapy of human tumour xenografts overexpressing the EGF receptor with rat antibodies that block the growth factor-receptor interaction. *British Journal of Cancer* **67**: 254–261.

Moghal N, Sternberg PW (1999) Multiple positive and negative regulators of signalling by the EGF receptor. *Current Opinions in Cell Biology* **11**: 190–196.

Nakagawa K, Yamamoto N, Kudoh S et al. (2000) A phase I intermittent dose-escalation trial of ZD1839 (Iressa) in Japanese patients with solid tumours. *Proceedings of the American Society of Clinical Oncology* **19**: 711 (abstract).

Negoro S, Nakagawa K, Fukuoka M et al. (2001) Final results of a phase I intermittent dose-escalation trial of ZD1839 (Iressa) in Japanese patients with various solid tumours. *Proceedings of the American Society of Clinical Oncology* **20**: 1292 (abstract).

Olapade-Olaopa EO, Moscatello DK, MacKay EH et al. (2000) Evidence for the differential expression of a variant EGF receptor protein in human prostate cancer. *British Journal of Cancer* **82**: 186–192.

Perrotte P, Matsumoto T, Inoue K et al. (1999) Anti-epidermal growth factor receptor antibody C225 inhibits angiogenesis in human transitional cell carcinoma growing orthotopically in nude mice. *Clinical Cancer Research* **5**: 257–265.

Pravelic K, Banjac Z, Pavelic J et al. (1993) Evidence for a role of EGF receptor in the progression of human lung carcinoma. *Anticancer Research* **13**: 1133–1137.

Prenzel N, Zwick E, Daub H et al. (1999) EGF receptor transactivation by G-protein coupled receptors requires metalloproteinase cleavage of proHB-EGF. *Nature* **402**: 884–888.

Prenzel N, Zwick E, Leserer M, Ulrich A (2000) Tyrosine kinase signalling in breast cancer: epidermal growth factor receptor: convergence point for signal integration and diversification. *Breast Cancer Research Treat* **2**: 184–190.

Prewett M, Rockwell P, Rose C, Goldstein NI (1996) Anti-tumour and cell cycle responses in KB cells treated with a chimeric anti-EGFR monoclonal antibody in combination with cisplatin. *International Journal of Cancer* **9**: 217–224.

Raben D, Buchsbaum DJ, Gillespie Y et al. (1999) Treatment of human intracranial gliomas with chimeric monoclonal antibody against the epidermal growth factor receptor in creases the survival of nude mice when treated concurrently with radiotherapy. *Proceedings of the American Association of Cancer Research* **40**: 1244 (abstract).

Rao GS, Ethier SP (1999) Potentiation of radiation induced breast cancer cell death by inhibition of epidermal growth factor family of receptors. *International Journal of Radiation Biology* **45**(suppl): 162.

Rodek U, Herlyn M, Herlyn D et al. (1987) Tumour growth modulation by a monoclonal antibody to the epidermal growth factor receptor: immunologically mediated and effector cell-independent effects. *Cancer Research* **47**: 3692–3696.

Rusch V, Klimasta D, Venatraman E et al. (1997) Overexpression of the epidermal growth factor receptor and its ligand transforming growth factor alpha is frequent in resectable non-small cell lung cancer but does not predict tumour progression. *Clinical Cancer Research* **37**: 515–522.

Salomon DS, Brandt R, Ciardiello F et al. (1995) Epidermal growth factor-related peptides and their receptors in human malignancies. *Critical Review of Oncology/Haematology* **19**: 183–232.

Sato JD, Kawamoto J, Le A et al. (1983) Biological effects in vitro of monoclonal antibodies to human epidermal growth factor receptor. *Molecular Biology and Medicine* **1**: 511–529.

Schmidt M, Wels W (1996) Targeted inhibition of tumour cell growth by a bi-specific single-chain toxin containing an antibody domain and TGFα. *British Journal of Cancer* **74**: 853–862.

Schreiber AB, Winkler ME, Derynck R (1986) Transforming growth factor alpha: a more potent angiogenic mediator than epidermal growth factor. *Science* **232**: 1250–1253.

Sunada H, Magun BE, Mendelsohn J, MacLeod CL (1986) Monoclonal antibody against epidermal growth factor receptor is internalised without stimulation receptor phosphorylation. *Proceedings of the National Academy of Science of the USA* **83**: 3825–3829.

Trumell HQ, Raish B, Ahmed A et al. (1999) The biologic effects of anti-epidermal growth factor receptor and ionising radiation in human head and neck tumour cell lines. *Proceedings of the American Association of Cancer Research* **40**: 958 (abstract).

Veale D, Kerr N, Gibson GJ et al. (1993) The relationship of quantitative epidermal growth factor receptor expression in non-small cell lung cancer to long term survival. *British Journal of Cancer* **68**: 162–165.

Velu TJ (1990) Structure, function and transforming potential of the epidermal growth factor receptor. *Molecular and Cellular Endocrinology* **70**: 205–216

Viloria Petit AM, Rak J, Hung MC et al. (1997) Neutralising antibodies against epidermal growth factor and ErB-2/neu receptor tyrosine kinases down regulate vascular endothelial cell growth factor production by tumour cells in vitro and in vivo. *American Journal of Pathology* **151**: 1523–1530.

Voldborg BR, Damstrup L, Sprang-Thomsen M et al. (1997) Epidermal growth factor receptor (EGFR) and EGFR mutations, function and possible role in clinical trials *Annals of Oncology* **8**: 1197–1206.

Volm M, Rittgen W, Drings P (1998) Prognostic value of ERBB-1, VEGF, cyclin A, FOS, JUN and MYC in patients with squamous cell lung carcinomas. *British Journal of Cancer* **77**: 663–669.

Wen X, Li C, Wu Q-P et al. (2000a) Potentiation of antitumour activity of PG-TXL with anti EGFR monoclonal antibody C225 in MDA-MB-468 human breast cancer xenograft. *Proceedings of the American Association of Cancer Research* **41**: 2052 (abstract).

Wen X, Li C, Wu QP et al. (2000b) Potentiation of the antitumour activity of PG-TXL with anti-EGFR monoclonal antibody C225 in MDA-MB-468 human breast cancer xenograft. *Proceedings of the American Association of Cancer Research* **41**: 2052 (abstract).

Wikstrand CJ, hale LP, Batra SK et al. (1995) monoclonal antibodies against EGFRvIII are tumour specific and react with breast and lung carcinomas and malignant gliomas. *Cancer Research* **55**: 3140–3148.

Wikstrand CJ, McLendon RE, Friedman AH et al. (1997) Cell surface localization and density of the tumour associated variant of the epidermal growth factor receptor, EGFRvIII. *Cancer Research* **57**: 4130–4140.

Woodburn JR (1999) The epidermal growth factor receptor and its inhibition in cancer therapy. *Pharmacology and Therapeutics* **82**: 241–250.

Yamauchi T, Ueki K, Tobe K et al. (1997) Tyrosine phosphorylation of the EGF receptor by the kinase Jak2 is induced by growth hormone. *Nature* **390**: 91–96.

PART 5

Clinical governance

Guidance on the management of lung cancer issued by NICE and the demand for chemotherapy in NSCLC

Michael Cullen

In 1998, the EUROCARE project reported on survival outcomes for major tumour types across Europe (Coebergh et al. 1998). The figures showed that lung cancer patients in the UK lived shorter lives than those in much of mainland Europe. Expert meetings were held to examine these alarming findings in case they were artefactual and merely the result of different standards with the countries with the best outcomes having the most population-based complete data. Regrettably, no alternative explanation emerged and the inescapable conclusion was that treatment of lung and some other common cancers in the UK was seriously suboptimal. This raised something of a political storm and led to the appointment of a National Cancer Director and the production of the NHS Cancer Plan (Department of Health 2000).

Lung cancer management problems in the UK

There are a number of possible reasons for the poor outcomes of lung cancer management in this country. The EUROCARE report cited possibilities, including a shortage of lung cancer specialists and poorer access to specialised care. More specifically, a low rate of histological diagnosis almost certainly attests to a lack of clinical rigour in the management of lung cancer patients in the UK (Table 9.1).

The main effect of failure to secure a precise histological diagnosis is consequent failure to consider appropriate treatment. The most serious result is the omission of surgery in potentially curable patients. In 1998–99, 3711 thoracotomies for lung cancer were performed in the UK, which is about 10% of all lung cancer patients. In Rotterdam the equivalent regional registry-based figure is exactly double this (Damhuis and Schutte 1996). There is little doubt that we perform fewer potentially curative resections for lung cancer in this country compared with elsewhere.

The delivery of radiotherapy is little better. Despite UK-generated evidence for the greater efficacy of continuous hyperfractionated accelerated radiotherapy (CHART) in localised, inoperable non-small cell lung cancer (NSCLC), very few centres are able to deliver this treatment. Unacceptable delays in commencing radical radiotherapy are also widespread (O'Rourke and Edwards 2000).

The use of chemotherapy in NSCLC differs widely and is estimated to vary between 5% and 20% of patients with NSCLC. Clearly not all patients with the disease should be considered for chemotherapy, but there is a real difficulty in knowing what is the correct proportion. Relying on estimates based on diagnosed referrals to multidisciplinary teams risks missing an unknown proportion who may be diagnosed histologically and not referred, as well as those not diagnosed in the first place. As part of a publication describing their role, The Royal College of Physicians' Joint Specialty Committee (RCP 2000) for Medical Oncology attempted to predict the future requirement for medical oncologists by estimating the proportion of cancer patients within the population who might reasonably be considered for chemotherapy at some time in their lives.

The potential demand for chemotherapy in lung cancer in England and Wales

There are over 37 000 cases of lung cancer annually in England and Wales (Office of National Statistics 1992). In the Yorkshire Lung Cancer Referral Patterns audit of 1999 (Northern and Yorkshire Cancer Registry and Information Service [NYCRIS] 1999), 12% of these were histologically diagnosed as small cell lung cancer (SCLC). All others are treated as NSCLC, including those without histological diagnosis. Decisions concerning the applicability of chemotherapy depend critically on performance status (PS) and stage. Population-based statistics for age distribution within different cancers are available, but those for PS are harder to find. There are, nevertheless, some published data based on prospective audits. Where PS data are not available estimates have been used. Age cut-offs for chemotherapy are inevitably arbitrary, but have been set at levels where it is thought that as many patients below a given age will not be suitable for chemotherapy as there are above who will.

For SCLC patients, 80 years is selected as the age cut-off and PS distributions (ambulatory 0, 1, 2 vs non-ambulatory 3, 4) are estimated. Thus, 12% of all lung cancers are SCLC and just over 60% are aged 80 or less with performance status 0, 1 or 2, and hence are eligible for consideration for chemotherapy. This represents 2733 cases of SCLC, or 61% of the total. Two population-based audits of chemotherapy usage in SCLC are available, from Scotland (Gregor et al. 1999) and Yorkshire (NYCRIS 1999). In Scotland in 1995, 61% of 681 patients received chemotherapy, and in Yorkshire between 1986 and 1994 55% did so. There has been little change in the perceived role of chemotherapy in this disease in the last 15 years, and the remarkable similarity between the estimated and actual figures attests to the validity of the estimations.

According to the UK Society of Cardiothoracic Surgeons, 10% of cases of NSCLC are resected and 63% of these will fail. An estimated 25% of these will be of poor PS, leaving about 1500 operated cases eligible for chemotherapy. The vast majority of NSCLC cases are inoperable. A small proportion has well-localised, inoperable disease and are candidates for radical radiotherapy. However, the BMJ meta-analysis of 1995 (Non-small Cell Lung Cancer Collaborative Group 1995) showed that survival was better when radiotherapy was preceded by chemotherapy for these, as well as for patients with more advanced stages.

In the Yorkshire Lung Cancer Referral Patterns audit, 73.5% of lung cancer patients had a bronchoscopy and the RCP bronchoscopy audit of 1680 patients in 1999 did prospectively document PS (NYCRIS 1999). A higher proportion of operable cases is likely to have had bronchoscopy and so the 73.5% figure has been recalculated, assuming that all operable cases had a bronchoscopy. The proportion in advanced disease then becomes 70.5%; 10% of these were PS 3 or 4, leaving 18 749 patients of good PS who underwent bronchoscopy. Using an age cut-off of 75 (the upper age limit for most, but not all, randomised trials – demonstrating benefit from chemotherapy in advanced NSCLC), this produces 13 500 patients eligible for consideration of chemotherapy. The patients who did not undergo bronchoscopy are a mix of poor PS cases and cases diagnosed in other ways (pleural cytology, node biopsy, etc.). Assuming a 75 : 25 split between these, and the same 75-year cut-off, a further 1286 cases are eligible. The total is 16 337, or 50% of all cases of NSCLC. In their assessment of the new chemotherapeutic agents available for this disease (see below), the National Institute for Clinical Excellence (NICE) accepted that currently only 5–20% of cases were receiving chemotherapy.

Effective systemic treatment has existed for several years now with good evidence for survival prolongation in advanced disease and palliation (Cullen et al. 1999). The four drugs docetaxel, paclitaxel, gemcitabine and vinorelbine are likely to be more convenient than existing therapies but may not be more effective.

NICE process and guidance

In August 2000, the Department of Health asked NICE to review the four drugs docetaxel, paclitaxel, gemcitabine and vinorelbine in the context of advanced NSCLC. In turn, NICE commissioned the assessment report, invited submissions from interested groups including The Royal Colleges, cancer charities, the pharmaceutical industry, patient groups, etc., and appointed external independent experts.

The assessment report was commissioned from the Wessex Institute for Health Research and Development Rapid Reviews team. Sponsor submissions came from Aventis Pharma Ltd, BMS Pharmaceuticals Ltd, Eli Lilly & Co Ltd and Pierre Fabre Ltd. Professional submissions came from the Joint Collegiate Council for Oncology (JCCO) and The Royal College of General Practitioners. Patient group submissions were received from CancerBACUP, Macmillan Cancer Relief and the Roy Castle Lung Cancer Foundation. The patient advocates invited to the NICE appraisal committee for this project were Judith Brodie and Jesme Baird, while the experts were Penella Woll and the author. The NICE appraisal committee members included 12 academics with backgrounds in clinical pharmacology (two), morbid anatomy, general practice, gastroenterology, nephrology, diabetes, community practice development, public health, health economics (two) and health-related research. There were three trust, health authority, or primary care group executives, a charity chief executive and a former executive director of the National Council for Hospices/Palliative Care Services. There were four clinical NHS employees including a consultant surgeon and two GPs, a statistician and a pharmaceutical industry representative.

The Appraisal Committee agenda began with declaration of interests and then there was a presentation by the Wessex review group. There was time for members of the committee to question the experts and patient advocates. A number of misunderstandings about palliative chemotherapy were clarified. In practice, most patients do not receive the maximum number of cycles of palliative chemotherapy because assessments are (or certainly should be) made with every cycle to determine benefit. Patients should proceed beyond a single cycle only if symptomatic improvement accrues (with good tolerance of treatment), and beyond two cycles only if both symptomatic and objective (generally chest radiograph response) benefit results.

Following the appraisal committee meeting, the provisional appraisal determination is circulated for consultation, amended, and then released to the NHS and the general public. For future appraisals NICE have agreed to involve the nominated experts much earlier on in the process.

Table 9.1 Histological verification rates for lung cancer in Europe as reported in the EUROCARE II study for 1985–9 (and UK Clinical Outcome Guidance recommendations)

Lung cancer (% histological verification)	1985–1989	EUROCARE II 1998
England 1985–89	58%	
Scotland 1995	61%	
Finland	91%	
Denmark	88%	
Slovenia	87%	
Estonia	69%	
Netherlands, Austria, Germany, France, Spain, Italy, Switzerland	72–99%	< 20% national population covered for these
UK COG guidelines	Min. 70%	[11]

Conclusions

Summarised above is evidence that lung cancer is often inadequately investigated and treated in the UK. The evidence cited includes a low rate of histological verification, surgical resection, optimal radiotherapy, chemotherapy utilisation and survival relative to other developed countries. The reasons for this may be:

- ignorance about the disease and what can be achieved with optimal treatment
- prejudice among some professional groups against active intervention
- the perceived and actual cost of optimal treatment
- shortage of sufficient radiotherapy equipment
- low numbers of dedicated lung cancer surgeons, oncologists, specialist nurses and radiographers
- a system that, until recently, was not conducive to multidisciplinary decision-making
- a notoriously undemanding, unassertive patient population.

Reviewing the data NICE concluded that chemotherapy (supervised by appropriately trained and experienced professionals) should be considered in patients who are unsuitable for curative treatment, and that paclitaxel, gemcitabine or vinorelbine plus a platinum drug are recommended for first-line treatment and docetaxel should be considered when relapse has occurred after prior chemotherapy (NICE 2001). The guidance document estimates that currently 5–20% of patients with unresectable NSCLC are offered chemotherapy. Using the best data available the RCP Committee for Medical Oncology has shown that as many as 50% of cases should be considered for chemotherapy during at least one stage in the natural history of the disease. Clearly there needs to be major reforms in the way we think about managing lung cancer in this country, as well as resource enhancements to ensure that optimum care is delivered to a relatively deprived patient population.

References

Coebergh J, Sant M, Berrino F, Verdecchia A (1998) Survival of adult cancer patients in Europe diagnosed from 1978–1989: The Eurocare II Study. *European Journal of Cancer* **34**: 2137–2278.

Cullen MH, Billingham LJ, Woodroffe C et al. (1999) MIC in unresectable NSCLC: effects on survival and quality of life. *Journal of Clinical Oncology* **17**: 3188–3194.

Damhuis RA, Schutte PR (1996) Resection rates and postoperative mortality in 7899 patients with lung cancer. *European Respiratory Journal* **9**: 7–10.

Department of Health (2000) *The NHS Cancer Plan: A plan for investment, a plan for reform.* London: DoH.

Gregor A, Stroner PL, Davidson J, Thomson CS (1999) Lung cancer in Scotland – The 1995 reality. *British Journal of Cancer* **80**(suppl 2): 15.

National Institute for Clinical Excellence (2001) *Guidance on the Use of Docetaxel, Paclitaxel, Gemcitabine and Vinorelbine for the Treatment of Non-small Cell Lung Cancer.* London: NICE.

NHS Executive (1998) *Guidance on Commissioning Cancer Services. Improving outcomes in lung cancer.* London: NHS Executive.

Non-small Cell Lung Cancer Collaborative Group (1995) Chemotherapy in non-small cell lung cancer: a meta-analysis using updated data on individual patients from 52 randomised trials. *British Medical Journal* **311**: 899–909.

Northern and Yorkshire Cancer Registry and Information Service (NYCRIS) (1999) *Cancer Treatment Policies and Their Effects on Survival. Key Sites Study 2. Lung.* Leeds: NYCRIS.

Office of National Statistics (1992) *Cancer Incidence Data for England and Wales.* London: The Stationery Office.

O'Rourke N, Edwards R (2000) Lung cancer treatment waiting times and tumour growth. *Clinical Oncology* **12**: 141–144.

Royal College of Physicians (2000) *The Cancer Patient's Physician: Recommendations for the development of medical oncology in England and Wales.* London: RCP.

The Manual NHS Exec. (1998) Guidance on commissioning cancer services. Improving outcomes in lung cancer.

Chapter 10

Developing lung cancer services – the impact of modernisation of the NHS

RJ Fergusson and Anna Gregor

Lung cancer remains the major cause of death from malignant disease in the Western World. Almost 40 000 people are diagnosed with primary lung cancer in the UK every year and, although the incidence of the condition is gradually falling in men, it is becoming more common in women and, as a cause of death, has overtaken breast cancer in many parts of the country. The prognosis of lung cancer patients is extremely poor. Approximately 5% remain alive for 5 years after diagnosis and survival prospects have changed little in the last two or three decades. Comparisons with survival rates reported by some other European countries have caused much attention in the last few years (Janssen-Heijnen et al. 1998) (Figure 10.1).

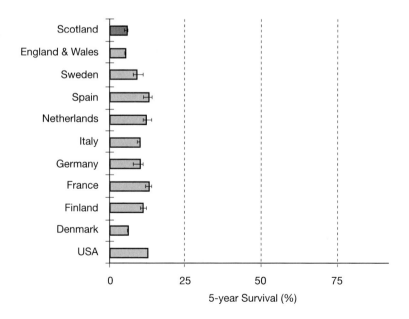

Figure 10.1 Lung cancer: 5-year survival.

There are a number of possible reasons why survival from lung cancer in the UK appears poorer than our European neighbours, including the following:

- Late presentation of patients with advanced stage disease
- Significant co-morbidity (ischaemic heart disease, peripheral vascular disease and chronic obstructive airway disease)
- Delays in investigation and treatment
- Lack of specialist involvement at all stages in the patient's cancer journey
- Exclusion of patients from investigation and treatment on the basis of age (Brown et al. 1996)
- Therapeutic nihilism by clinicians withholding treatment from potentially treatable patients
- More complete cancer registration data giving apparently lower survival percentages.

It is likely that a number of the above factors do operate and explain the gulf between lung cancer survival in the UK and in other Westernised societies. Recently reported population-based studies using cancer registry data in the UK (Northern and Yorkshire Cancer Registry and Information Service [NYCRIS] 1999; Gregor et al. 2001) have shown poor uptake of treatments known to prolong survival and marked geographical variations in investigations, waiting times and access to specific anti-cancer therapies. However, these data were collected at a time before the publication of nationally agreed lung cancer management guidelines (British Thoracic Society [BTS] 1998; NHS Executive 1998; Scottish Intercollegiate Guidelines Network [SIGN] 1998; Royal College of Radiologists' COIN 1999).

In Scotland in 1995, three-quarters of patients registered with lung cancer had a definitive histological diagnosis and a similar number were assessed by a respiratory physician (Gregor et al. 2001). However, only just over half received some form of active therapy (surgery 10.7%, radiotherapy 35.8%, chemotherapy 16.1%). Survival was poor (median 3.6 months) with 21.1% only alive at 1 year and 7% at 3 years.

To try to address the obvious inequalities of care for patients with cancer in general, the government has launched *The National Cancer Plan* (NHS Executive 2000) and in Scotland a similar document *Cancer in Scotland – Action for Change* (Scotish Executive 2001) has also appeared. Both initiatives have been accompanied by a significant increase in Exchequer funding in an attempt to implement the ideals outlined in the strategies. What changes are proposed in the Scottish document and are they likely to improve the effectiveness of lung cancer services in the future?

Cancer in Scotland – action for change

This 63-page document outlines the current status of cancer treatment in Scotland and puts in place proposals for developing services in a number of areas. Cancer prevention, early detection, access to diagnosis and therapy, palliative care, and research and technology issues are all covered. The cornerstone of the new cancer services is the delivery of care by managed clinical networks (MCNs) working through regional cancer advisory groups. These will be situated in the west, south-east and north of Scotland. Standards of care are to be continuously monitored and improved locally and nationally using the already established Clinical Standards Board for Scotland (CSBS) which has been developed over the last 2 years.

Managed clinical networks in lung cancer

The Calman–Hine model for the management of cancer patients while being adopted in England and Wales did not lend itself well to Scotland's geographical layout. The Scottish Executive, therefore, has turned to MCNs as a model for the management of the common cancers (Scottish Executive 1999). These networks comprise groups of multidisciplinary professionals working in a particular field who look after patients with a specific tumour type. A successful network depends on clinicians agreeing to treat patients using set clinical protocols, which are usually agreed on a local and national level. The group should continuously collect prospective data about the patient's journey and the outcomes of treatment; these data should be regularly shared between members of the group. This allows clinicians to run a local service to a prescribed standard and will identify clinical practice that may be regarded as idiosyncratic. The boundaries of MCNs are not usually those of health boards and trusts. It is anticipated that the MCNs in Scotland will be set up under the auspices of three regional cancer advisory groups (north, west and south-east Scotland), each providing a strategic advisory and planning focus for their respective locality cancer services and NHS boards.

South-East Scotland Cancer Network

Cancer professionals in south-east Scotland had been working together for a number of years to provide coordinated clinical care across a range of services and geographical areas. What was not available was a systematic quality assurance programme and formal management links to the NHS and to voluntary organisations providing different parts of the service. In April 2000 the South-East Scotland Cancer Network (SCAN) was set up by the collaboration of four health boards in the region (Fife, Lothian, Borders, and Dumfries and Galloway). This 'virtual' organisation now has managerial support and has developed managed clinical networks in the four common cancers (breast, lung, colorectal and gynaecological).

The SCAN lung group evolved from the South-East of Scotland Lung Cancer Group, which had a record of data collection and audit in the past (Fergusson et al.

1996). It covers a population of approximately 1.2 million with patients being referred to six separate respiratory units (four district general hospital and two university teaching hospitals). Treatment is carried out in the thoracic surgical unit and the regional radiotherapy department in the two respective teaching hospitals. Chemotherapy is also given locally in two of the four district general hospitals. The lung group is truly multiprofessional (Table 10.1) and has met at regular intervals over the last 2 years. The group has agreed to adopt national lung cancer guidelines (SIGN) and has collected data concerning its patients prospectively since its inception. The group has just begun to compare data over the last year (to October 2000). Case ascertainment has been approximately 80% of numbers appearing on the Scottish Cancer Registry. Significant differences between waiting times for investigations and treatment have once again been observed. The group has been able to make direct comparison of local management arrangements between individual hospitals. This has allowed planning of a more uniform service across south-east Scotland and will hopefully allow a more equitable access of patients to investigations and treatment.

Table 10.1 SCAN Lung Cancer Group members

Respiratory physicians	Primary care physicians
Thoracic surgeons	Specialist nurses
Radiation oncologists	Patient representatives
Medical oncologists	Audit facilitators
Radiologists	Pharmacists
Pathologists	Management representatives

Clinical Standards Board for Scotland

The Clinical Standards Board for Scotland (CSBS) was established as a special health board in April 1999. Its remit was to develop and run a national system of quality assurance and accreditation of clinical services. The Board defined standards for clinical services and has assessed performance throughout the NHS in Scotland against these standards. The four common cancers were initially selected as a national clinical priority. A CSBS lung cancer project group was convened in January 2000 and produced draft clinical standards for lung cancer within 3 months. After an open meeting and consultation period, a modified version of the standards was piloted at three trusts across Scotland in July 2000. The final standards for lung cancer were published in January 2001. The evidence base for the clinical standards for lung cancer was principally drawn from the SIGN lung cancer guidelines (1998) and covers all aspects of the patient's lung cancer journey (Table 10.2).

Table 10.2 Clinical Standards Board for Scotland (lung cancer standards)

Referral process	Management
Investigations	Surgery
Multidisciplinary working	Radiotherapy
Education and training	Chemotherapy
Audit	Symptom management
Clinical trials	Drugs
Communication	Equipment
Assessment/care plans	

Throughout 2001 all the acute trusts in Scotland have had their lung cancer service assessed by external peer review. These evaluations were based on an objective assessment of written evidence from each trust and a visit by a small multidisciplinary team to the locations where the service was provided. Each review team included lay members as well as clinicians, nurses and paramedics involved on a daily basis with lung cancer patients. In March 2002, the CSBS published a report providing a national assessment of performance against the standards that it has set. This highlights where clinical performance has fallen below standards and makes suggestions for quality improvements. It is also an opportunity to disseminate good practice where standards have been exceeded. This model of quality assurance of clinical services would appear to be unique in the Western World and a number of European countries are considering adopting a similar model.

Conclusions

Patients with lung cancer in the UK appear to fare worse than their European counterparts. The reasons for this are not clear but are likely to include inequalities in access to effective anti-cancer treatments. In 2001 the British government has introduced strategic plans and investments to improve cancer services. In Scotland, these developments include a central role for MCNs and a system of peer review and accreditation of lung cancer services. It is hoped that this modernisation of lung cancer services will translate into improved outcomes for lung cancer patients.

References

British Thoracic Society Standards of Care Committee, Lung Cancer Working Party (1998) BTS recommendations to respiratory physicians for organising the care of patients with lung cancer. *Thorax* **53**(suppl 1): S1–S8.

Brown JS, Erraut D, Trask C, Davidson AG (1996) Age and the treatment of lung cancer. *Thorax* **51**: 564–568.

Clinical Standards Board for Scotland (2002) *Lung Cancer Services*. Edinburgh: CSBS.

Fergusson RJ, Gregor A, Dodds R, Kerr G (1996) Management of lung cancer in South-East Scotland. *Thorax* **51**: 569–574.

Gregor A, Thomson CS, Brewster DH et al. (2001) Management and survival of lung cancer patients diagnosed in 1995 in Scotland: results of a national population-based study. *Thorax* **56**: 212–217.

Janssen-Heijnen MLG, Gatta G, Forman D, Capocaccia R, Coebergh JWW and the EUROCARE Working Group (1998) Variation in survival of patients with lung cancer in Europe, 1985–1989. *European Journal of Cancer* **34**: 2191–2196.

NHS Executive (1998) *Guidance on Commissioning Cancer Services: Improving outcomes in lung cancer – The Manual*. Leeds: Department of Health.

NHS Executive (2000) *The National Cancer Plan. A plan for investment, a plan for reform*. London: Department of Health.

Northern and Yorkshire Cancer Registry and Information Service (NYCRIS) (1999) *Cancer Treatment Policies and Their Effects on Survival. Key Sites Study 2. Lung*. Leeds: NYCRIS.

Royal College of Radiologists' Clinical Oncology Information Network (COIN) (1999) Guidelines on the non-surgical management of lung cancer. *Clinical Oncology* **11**: S1–S53.

Scottish Executive (1999) *Introduction of Managed Clinical Networks within the NHS in Scotland*. NHS Mel 10. Edinburgh: Scottish Executive Health Department.

Scottish Executive (2001) *Cancer in Scotland. Action for change*. Edinburgh: Scottish Executive Health Department.

Scottish Intercollegiate Guidelines Network (1998) *Management of Lung Cancer*, No 23. Edinburgh: SIGN.

Chapter 11

The impact of lung cancer patient groups on the delivery of the clinical service

Jesme Baird

This chapter examines the emerging role and the potential impact of lung cancer patients in influencing and improving the quality of lung cancer service provision. Breast cancer and HIV patient groups, in particular, have shown that patients can be successful in raising awareness, improving disease profiles, increasing funding and altering clinical services. To date, there has been little mobilisation of lung cancer patients in this respect because, in other disease areas, it has been the voluntary sector that has coordinated patients for this purpose. This is, however, perhaps not surprising, because there are only two lung cancer-specific voluntary organisations in the world – the Alliance for Lung Cancer Advocacy Support and Education in the USA and the Roy Castle Lung Cancer Foundation in the UK.

Individual case studies and specific examples support the positive influence that patients, in general, can exert. There is, however, a clear lack of information and evidence-based research to support the most effective strategies in achieving this.

There are two main ways in which patients can have an impact on clinical service provision:

1. By direct involvement in the process itself, so called 'user involvement'.
2. By exerting external pressure for service change and improvement, through media campaigning and political lobbying.

User involvement in cancer services

The publication by the Department of Health, in 1995, of *A Policy Framework for Commissioning Cancer Services* paved the way for cancer patient involvement in service provision, by recommending that services be 'patient centred'.

Since then, user involvement has been highlighted in many subsequent Department of Health planning documentation, throughout the UK – *The NHS Plan* (DoH 2000a), *National Cancer Plan: A Plan for Investment: A Plan for Reform* (DoH 2000b), *Cancer Information Strategy* (DoH 2000c), *Cancer in Scotland: Action for Change* (Scottish Executive Health Department 2001).

There is a lack of research evidence in this field. Avon, Somerset and Wiltshire Cancer Services has been awarded a grant through the Department of Health's Health in Partnership initiative to develop and evaluate best practice for user involvement in cancer services. This project is expected to run until autumn 2002.

Presently, however, no guidance exists on how meaningful cancer patient participation can be achieved. Thus, user involvement has developed on an ad hoc basis within cancer networks, using various methods to involve patients in service provision (Bradburn 2001), namely:

• Patient consultation through surveys and questionnaires or through patient focus groups.
• Active partnership with user representatives as members of committees or working groups.

Achieving effective user representation

There are a number of benefits from actively involving patients in developing services:

• in supporting and motivating health professionals to provide high-quality services
• in ensuring that services reflect the reality for people using them, thereby improving quality
• in demonstrating that the experiences of service users are valued
• in developing a shared responsibility for health
• in promoting openness and accountability.

There is clear evidence that people affected with cancer, in general, both have the ability and are willing to have a voice and make a contribution by highlighting areas for improvement (National Cancer Alliance 1996; Walker et al. 1996). However, as with the 1996 National Cancer Alliance study, research projects investigating cancer patients in general tend to be biased towards breast cancer patients in particular. In this particular project, 33 of the 75 patients in the study had breast cancer, and only one, lung cancer.

Several comprehensive reports on the patterns of lung cancer service provision and treatment have been compiled in the UK in recent years (Standing Medical Advisory Committee 1994; British Thoracic Society 1998; NHS Executive 1998; Scottish Intercollegiate Guidelines Network 1998). These provide expert recommendations for treatment patterns and future service developments. They offer little insight, however, into the experiences and needs of patients and families living with a diagnosis of lung cancer. Patients with lung cancer have been shown to experience greater levels of unmet psychological, social and economic needs than other cancer groups (Houts et al. 1986). They have also been shown to be less satisfied with their care than other people who have cancer (Fakhoury et al. 1997). A national needs assessment of lung cancer patients and their carers, undertaken on behalf of Macmillan Cancer Relief, identified a myriad of deficiencies in the delivery of care, in information, and support (Krishnasamy and Wilkie 1999). It is, therefore, important for lung cancer patients themselves to be involved in the service planning process.

Lung cancer and user representation

Although the most common cancer diagnosis in the UK, with around 40 000 new cases each year (CRC Statistics 1999), there are currently very few lung cancer patient representatives involved in service planning and delivery.

Undoubtedly, there are, a number of inherent barriers to such patient involvement. With a median survival of 4 months from diagnosis, 80% of patients dead at 1 year and only around 5% surviving 5 years (NHS Centre for Reviews and Dissemination 1998), the average lung cancer patient may not survive the length of the working group. Furthermore, as most people with lung cancer are not only elderly, but also less fit than their contemporaries and often suffering from smoking-related illnesses, they may be too ill to attend meetings.

The pool for lung cancer patient representatives is therefore from the small group of long-term survivors. In the main, these will have presented with early stage disease and have been treated surgically. The experience of this group is considerably different from that of the majority. Thus, the issue of training becomes important.

Despite their willingness, there is, however, obvious concern about an individual patient's ability to represent a broad range of views, rather than his or her own individual experience – good or bad. This can be overcome by focus groups, to obtain the service user's views and recruit from these to the committee or working group (Beresford 2001). Of vital importance, therefore, is the selection of an appropriate, suitably knowledgeable patient representative to make a meaningful contribution.

Having an individual to represent the views of patients can overcome some of the lung cancer-specific issues. This individual can either be a relative/spouse/partner of a lung cancer patient or an independent representative, with specific knowledge of the lung cancer journey and meaningful contact with lung cancer patients. Increasingly, the latter is a role being taken by cancer voluntary sector organisations. Organisations historically dedicated to cancer patient support, through their contact with patients, are increasingly becoming involved with patient advocacy issues, e.g. the Roy Castle Lung Cancer Foundation's Patient Care Office.

There has, to date, been no systematic mapping of user involvement in cancer services in the UK. However, anecdotal comment suggests that, within cancer networks and on national committees and fora, for the reasons outlined above, lung cancer patient representatives are rare. In recent months, after multiple requests for user representatives from cancer networks and national bodies (e.g. the National Institute of Clinical Excellence, UK Co-ordinating Committee on Cancer Research [UKCCCR], Clinical Standards Board Scotland), the Roy Castle Lung Cancer Foundation has developed a system of providing an independent representative for such groups. These individuals have a sound knowledge of the lung cancer journey and meaningful contact with lung cancer patients, via the Foundation's Lung Cancer Patient Support Network. However, there are only a few such suitable individuals, with limited time.

Training

Service users, working with health professionals on committees, feel a lack of confidence, skill and understanding of medical jargon and the working structures of the NHS (Bradburn et al. 1999). Thus, isolated users on committees of health professionals have experienced significant difficulties in being actively involved. For meaningful input, patient representatives need to have a well-defined role within the committee or group, and the professional members need to acknowledge that the service user has a useful contribution to make.

In the USA, training courses have been specifically developed for lay representatives involved in cancer research – *Project Lead* and the *Patient Advocate Programme* of the American Association for Cancer Research. In the UK, members of the UKCCCR Consumer Liaison Committee have received some training in research methods.

Elsewhere in the UK, training courses are emerging for breast cancer representatives, within the work of the UK Breast Cancer Coalition and for generic cancer patient representatives involved in health service, through the *CancerVOICES* Project of the charity Cancerlink. No training has, as yet, been developed specifically for lung cancer patients.

Lung cancer patient representation – future direction

On 11 September 2001, the Roy Castle Lung Cancer Foundation held the first National Lung Cancer Patient Meeting in the UK. It was attended by over 70 lung cancer patients and carers. The main focus for the day was lung cancer patient advocacy. From this beginning, it is hoped that the already established framework of 15 local Roy Castle Lung Cancer Support Groups across the UK will begin to link more closely with local lung cancer clinicians. Under the direction of the Foundation, they will work in partnership with local health professionals, to help to ensure the provision of best practice services for all. In time and with adequate resources, perhaps the network of groups will cover every health authority area. Adequate resources and the endorsement and contribution of local clinicians are needed for success.

While developing a structure wherein lung cancer patients can contribute, it is similarly important to ensure that the contribution is meaningful. For this, it is important to answer the following questions:

- Who makes sure, within the committee or group, that the patient representative is not merely a 'tick the box'?
- Does anyone monitor the effects of patient representation and whether or not it has made a difference to service provision?

Exerting external pressure

External influences, such as public pressure and political pressure, can have a positive impact on service delivery. In breast cancer and HIV, patients and patient groups have been shown to be powerful agents in directing such pressure.

A sense of pessimism surrounds lung cancer, both within the professional community and among the general public. In a survey, carried out by MORI for the Cancer Research Campaign, published in December 2000, seven out of ten people in the UK said that lung cancer patients who smoked had brought the disease on themselves. These negative perceptions have undoubtedly influenced the ways in which patients with lung cancer are managed (NHS Executive 1998). Indeed, lung cancer is generally viewed, even by patients themselves, as a self-inflicted disease, with no hope of survival. Such negativity leads to barriers and delays in patient referral for diagnosis, treatment and care.

The media have the potential to reach many audiences from patients and the general public, to policy/decision-makers and politicians. However, lung cancer is often seen as a depressing disease, a sad story. For this reason, it is not considered newsworthy. This is mirrored in the relative underreporting of lung cancer in the media. Recent analysis of cancer media coverage in the USA (Blum et al. 2001) showed that lung cancer appeared in only 105 articles of the 600 analysed. Once smoking/tobacco stories were eliminated, only 9% of the coverage was lung cancer. This compared with 61% for breast cancer, 23% for prostate cancer and 17% for colorectal cancer.

Indeed, for such a common disease, lung cancer has a poor public profile. Messages of hope about prevention or surviving lung cancer appear least often in lung cancer stories, compared with other cancers (Blum et al. 2001). Without raising false hope, there is a need, therefore, to encourage survivor stories, to trumpet lung cancer research and new development, and to encourage a more positive view of the health improvements that can be achieved in lung cancer care.

To this end, through its Patient Support Network, the Roy Castle Foundation has developed a database of patients who are willing to talk to journalists and reporters about their disease. Although the numbers are currently small, they provide a source of human-interest information, valued by the media.

Raising lung cancer awareness and campaigning for change

Awareness campaigns have increasingly become important vehicles to engage the media and general public in becoming more educated and more aware about health issues (e.g. Pink Ribbon Month for Breast Cancer; Red Ribbons and HIV). Furthermore, raised awareness and higher profile have the obvious impact of concentrating the minds of health planners and politicians in prioritising diseases and services.

Learning from successful media strategies employed by organisations working in other disease areas, it is clear that a well-planned, well-represented and sustained media campaign would have the potential to bring about a positive change in attitude towards the negative perception of lung cancer among the general public.

Although other cancers, such as breast and colorectal cancer, have been promoted by a number of targeted high profile awareness events, lung cancer in the UK has had relatively few:

- Macmillan Cancer Relief's National Lung Cancer Campaign, launched in 1997, to highlight the importance of early diagnosis and general awareness of symptoms
- *Cancer Research Campaign Lung Cancer Month* in January 2001. Several press announcements during the month focused on CRC-funded lung cancer research work.
- Roy Castle Lung Cancer Foundation launch of '*Focus on Lung Cancer*' in March 2001, to raise awareness both about the potential of good quality care and about inequalities in research, treatment and care, and to campaign to have these addressed.

Exerting external pressure on lung cancer service provision – future developments

Two international initiatives to raise the profile of lung cancer were to begin in late 2001. First, for the past few years, the Alliance of Lung Cancer Advocacy, Support and Education (ALCASE) have facilitated a lung cancer awareness month in the USA, in November. This year, it is anticipated that their awareness pack will be distributed to more than 200 000 people, through events and through other contact organisations. In recognition of the international scale of this disease, November 2001 was to be designated Global Lung Cancer Awareness Month, with other countries becoming involved. It is hoped that UK organisations with an interest in lung cancer will contribute.

Second, a Global Lung Cancer Coalition was to launch in the autumn of 2001. Participating organisations, all with lung cancer patient contact, are from seven different countries. In drawing from the success of other disease campaigns, the Coalition aims to motivate both public support and also researchers and health policy groups to improve patient access to quality treatment and care. Its aims are to:

- place lung cancer squarely on the global health agenda
- lessen the stigma of lung cancer among patients, their families, their healthcare providers, policy-makers and the general public
- empower lung cancer patients and their loved ones to take a more active role in their care

- effect change in relevant legislative and regulatory policies, to optimise treatment and care of lung cancer patients.

At a national level, the Roy Castle Lung Cancer Foundation, with the endorsement and contribution of patients at the First National Lung Cancer Patient Meeting, will continue to strengthen its framework, whereby patients can meaningfully contribute to media work and to campaigning.

Conclusions

Currently, lung cancer patient group involvement in service planning and delivery is in its infancy. As yet, we do not know what impact patients will have. In other diseases, however, we have seen patients and patient groups successfully influence service delivery, both by direct involvement and by exerting external pressure, through campaigning and raising awareness.

Heath professionals, service planners, charities and patients are all committed to best practice. Patients can be a powerful voice in helping to achieve this. Patient involvement should be viewed as a constructive and collaborative way forward.

In the coming months, a number of structured initiatives will be launched, driven by voluntary sector lung cancer patient organisations. These will aim to increase the media profile of lung cancer, and to raise public awareness and encourage patient representatives to be involved in local services and national bodies. As with examples from other diseases, it will be difficult to assess the resultant impact made on service provision. Formal study is needed to ensure that patient involvement is meaningful. Ultimately, lung cancer services and outcomes will improve.

References

Beresford P (2001) *Palliative Care: Developing User Involvement, Improving Quality.* Report on the First National Seminar of Palliative Care Service Users and Workers. St Christopher's Education Centre, Sydenham. The Centre for Citizen Participation, Brunel University, Middlesex.

Blum D, Kennedy, VN, Boerckel W, Rieger PT (2001) Lung cancer – under-reported in the media. *Proceedings of the American Society of Clinical Oncology* **20**: abstract 1001.

Bradburn J, Fletcher G, Kennelly C (1999) *Voices in Action: Research Report.* London: College of Health.

Bradburn J (2001) *User Involvement in Cancer Services.* Report to the National Cancer Taskforce. London: Cancerlink.

British Thoracic Society (1998) British Thoracic Society recommendations to respiratory physicians for organising the care of patients with lung cancer. *Thorax* **53**: S1–S8.

Cancer Research Campaign (1999) *Cancerstatistics: Mortality – UK.* London: CRC.

Department of Health (1995) *Policy Framework for Commissioning Cancer Services: A Report by the Expert Advisory Group on Cancer to the Chief Medical Officers of England and Wales.* London: HMSO.

Department of Health (2000a) *The NHS Plan: A Plan for Investment: A Plan for Reform.* London: HMSO.

Department of Health (2000b) *National Cancer Plan: A Plan for Investment: A Plan for Reform*, London: HMSO.

Department of Health (2000c) *Cancer Information Strategy.* London: HMSO.

Fakhoury W, McCarthy M, Addington-Hall J (1997) The effects of the clinical characteristics of dying cancer patients on informal caregivers' satisfaction with palliative care. *Palliative Medicine* **11**: 107–115.

Houts P, Yasko J, Khan B, Schelzel G, Marcon K (1986) Unmet psychological, social and economic needs of persons with cancer in Pennsylvania. *Cancer* **58**: 2355–2361.

Krishnasamy M, Wilkie E (1999) Lung cancer: patient's and families' and professionals' perceptions of health care need. a national needs assessment study. Unpublished research report. London: Macmillan Practice Development Unit, Institute of Cancer Research.

National Cancer Alliance (1996) *'Patient-Centred Cancer Services?' – What Patients Say.* National Cancer Alliance.

NHS Executive (1998) *Guidance on Commissioning Cancer Services: Improving Outcomes in Lung Cancer – The Manual.* Leeds: Department of Health.

NHS Centre for Reviews and Dissemination, University of York (1998) Management of lung cancer. *Effective Health Care* **4**: 1–12.

Scottish Executive Health Department (2001) *Cancer in Scotland: Action for Change.* Edinburgh: The Stationery Office.

Scottish Intercollegiate Guidelines Network (1998) *Management of Lung Cancer.* Publication No. 23. Edinburgh: SIGN.

Standing Medical Advisory Committee (1994) *Management of Lung Cancer: Current Clinical Practices.* London: Department of Health.

Walker G, Bradburn J, Maher J (1996) *Breaking Bad News.* London: King's Fund.

Chapter 12

Auditing the quality of lung cancer services: towards formal accreditation and appraisal of clinical services

DR Baldwin

Clinical audit is an essential tool for monitoring the provision and quality of care for lung cancer patients. Observational studies have identified that there is significant variation in both provision and quality of services (Fergusson et al. 1996). The Calman–Hine report on Cancer Services, the British Thoracic Society, and the Standing Medical Advisory Committee have all identified the need for change in the management of lung cancer patients (Gilligan 1998). For clinical audit to take place there must be systematic measurement of predetermined data and a mechanism for defining areas for improvement followed by reassessment after changes (the audit cycle).

Recently, cancer audit has been facilitated by developments in information technology and re-structuring of cancer services. Calman–Hine recommendations have resulted in the formation of cancer networks that include an audit infrastructure, albeit insufficient at this time to collect comprehensive data. The cancer accreditation process has ensured that there is at least the necessary service infrastructure to provide minimum acceptable standards of care. It would seem appropriate that the next round of cancer accreditation will be asking more questions concerned with performance and hence audit will be necessary to provide that information. Various professional bodies have grasped the importance of having datasets that truly measure quality of clinical care and, therefore, are useful starting points for audit:

* *Information for Health* (Department of Health 1998)
* Cancer networks
* Cancer accreditation process
* Development of minimum datasets:

    - Royal College of Physicians
    - British Thoracic Society
    - Society of Cardiothoracic Surgeons of Great Britain and Northern Ireland
    - Royal College of Pathologists
    - Oncology datasets.

One such example is the development of the core dataset for lung cancer of The Royal College of Physicians. This has clear data definitions and is based on clinical care pathways (Thompson et al. 1999).

The Government white paper *Information for Health* sets out an ambitious plan for the development of information technology. In some respects the development of minimum datasets is a response to this and with improving information technology the facility to perform audit will be there (Department of Health 1998, 2001).

The challenge for clinicians

The positive developments summarised above should provide essential baseline information about the patient population, interventions and outcomes. Continuing audit provides successive information about the same categories. The information can then be matched to define standards given by available guidelines (NHS Executive 1998; Scottish Intercollegiate Guidelines Network 1998; Royal College of Radiologists' Clinical Oncology Information Network 1999). However, despite powerful driving forces for audit, a useful infrastructure and general agreement that audit is an essential tool, practical experience indicates that audit often provides exactly what is not wanted: incomplete information and inaccurate information. This can be very misleading and is arguably worse than collecting no data at all! Misinformation can lead to the inappropriate assumptions that changes are required when, in fact, they are not or can miss important deficiencies in clinical services. The challenge, then, for clinicians working with developing cancer services is to develop a robust, accurate and complete system for collecting agreed data that are to be used for audit.

Measuring quality – the essential tools

When thinking of audit tools, what often springs to mind is a paper-based questionnaire or data-collection form designed to provide information in the desired area. In reality the essential tools for auditing quality include more than just a carefully designed form. An audit form can include two of the essential tools. First, it provides a methodology for collecting data, although there are other methodologies that may not involve the use of audit forms. Second, it collects data and, therefore, provides a dataset of sorts that tends to be targeted to a specific area. For the audit form to be completed, there have to be personnel to collect the data – the third essential component for audit (and in reality one of the 'tools'). The last component, and the most important to the success of any audit, is that there is clinical sponsorship. The essential tools can be summarised as:

- Methodology: robust and sustainable
- Datasets: that truly reflect quality
- Personnel: all those involved in the clinical care pathway
- Clinical sponsorship: determined and sustained.

The methodology employed to collect data must be robust, to facilitate collection of those data and because data collection within a clinical service needs to be ongoing. However detailed a clinical audit is, if the methodology impairs the clinical service, then at best the audit will be partially completed initially with data collection gradually waning. Datasets must truly reflect measures of quality and, for this reason, they are appropriately being developed by clinicians who work at the coalface of clinical medicine. The problem with developing these datasets is often which data to include. The more one thinks about what one wants to know about patients and services, the greater the data. Figure 12.1 illustrates a useful concept of a pyramid structure for datasets. Pruning the amount of data analysed down to the absolute bare minimum can allow broad-brush comparisons between services in different geographical sites.

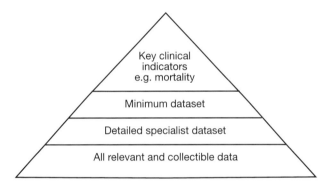

Figure 12.1 Datasets

In cancer services, the approach has been to collect six key clinical indicators based on wide discussion with clinicians involved in cancer care. The six key clinical indicators identified have been different for different tumour sites, but include items such as waiting times to initial consultation, waiting times to treatment, mortality, proportion seen by a multidisciplinary team, etc. However, if any differences are shown between sites, these key clinical indicators are insufficient to explain those differences and, therefore, they are included within the minimum (or 'core') dataset which should provide most of the information to explain the key clinical indicators. However, minimum datasets do not include certain essential data normally used in the course of clinical management. For this, a wider dataset is used which is termed here 'the detailed specialist dataset'. Beneath this are all collectable and relevant data. These data may not be essential to clinical management at all but, if specific questions are to be asked about a relatively small but potentially important part of the service, these data may need to be collected. An example might be a snapshot view of the patient's experience on the first visit to hospital using a detailed psychological evaluation. Inevitably, the development of minimum datasets will be an ongoing process with additions and deletions, refining them to achieve maximum relevance and efficiency.

Once the painstaking development of datasets, including clear and precise data definitions, has been completed, the first essential feature of good clinical data should have been achieved – relevance. The quality of clinical data from thereon depends on the methodology employed for collection. In addition, data must be accurate (and therefore verified), complete and easily accessible.

Personnel

In most existing clinical services data are collected, albeit in a written and relatively inaccessible form, by those who deal with the patient and by the patients themselves. It is, therefore, logical that in the setting of audit those same data should be collected, wherever possible, by all those involved in the clinical care pathway. As a result of potential impacts on clinical care imposed by the burden of data collection, methodology is again central to ensuring that data are collected.

Clinical sponsorship

Without doubt, the few areas where there is successful sustained collection of clinical audit and patient data have occurred where there is exemplary clinical sponsorship. Sponsorship has to be sustained and must provide crucial encouragement when the process falters. It is also an essential prerequisite to the development of methodology.

Methodology

Careful attention to methodology and clinical data collection is essential if the two pitfalls of data collection (incomplete data and inaccurate data) are to be avoided. Unfortunately it is all too often the case that 'technology [is] imposed before fundamental issues have been thought through' (Wyatt and Keen 2001). Details of methodology will necessarily vary depending on the clinical setting, but there are some essential common features that merit discussion. To illustrate some of these features we can turn to examples of good clinical data collection that have appeared in the literature. 'Real-time' data verification is one such essential component that minimises inaccurate data. This is facilitated by collecting data as an essential part of clinical management. The system of data collection is 'built in' to the service. Thus, if data collection is essential to management, these data will be accessed by the relevant healthcare professionals who are able to verify it. This is much more than simply ensuring 'double entry data'.

Inevitably when discussing information technology some consideration needs to be given to the software used. 'Clinician-sensitive software' is rarely found in medical information technology, but will in the future be an essential feature enabling the integration of data collection within the clinical service. Clinician-sensitive software should, where possible, resemble the usual clinical process and be as close to using a set of case notes as possible. If using a computer prolongs consultation time, this will almost certainly prevent integration with the service. This is largely because the 'rewards' from collecting data in health care are not sufficiently great to warrant prolongation of the clinical process. This is in contrast to the situation in industry. The third feature, therefore, of clinician-sensitive software is that it provides 'irresistible carrots' for the healthcare professional. This can be summarised as:

- It resembles the usual clinical process
- It does not prolong consultation
- It provides 'irresistible carrots'
- It must exploit new technologies in use in industry.

Examples of good clinical practice in cancer information technology

Although there are no published comprehensive real-time audit tools for lung cancer, there are examples of good practice and good clinical 'ideas'. If health information technology is to develop along the same lines as the worldwide web, then it will develop in a piecemeal fashion with gradual adoption of good practice, eventually leading to the full electronic health record. The first example (Taenzer et al. 2000) shows the effect of introducing a computerised quality-of-life screening tool and testing its effect on physician behaviour and patient satisfaction.

Figure 12.2 shows that lung cancer patients were divided into two groups: group 1 completed a computerised version of a quality-of-life questionnaire and group 2, to ensure that the same data were collected, completed the same questionnaire in a paper version after the clinic. The study showed that more quality-of-life issues were identified by the patient before the consultation in the first group and, as a consequence of this, more quality-of-life issues were addressed during the clinic appointment. This is an example of a system that can easily be introduced into lung cancer clinics and which provides, without any additional clinician effort and time, essential information. The study was not comprehensive in its assessment of the overall effect of introducing computerisation into the clinic setting. There are no examples of this sort of comprehensive evaluation in a lung oncology setting.

More detailed analyses have been performed in other settings. Our own work on the impact of computerisation on an asthma clinic gives some insight into the possible effects on patients (King et al. 1993). In this detailed analysis, a conventional asthma clinic was compared with one employing a paper-based audit tool and a fully

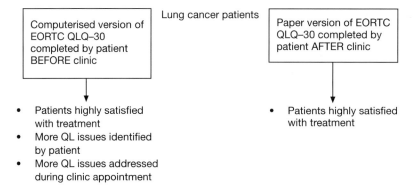

Figure 12.2 Computerised quality of life (QL) screening: effect on physician behaviour and patient satisfaction (Taenzer et al. 2000). EORTC, European Organisation for the Research and Treatment of Cancer.

computerised asthma clinic where patients entered their own morbidity data before consultation. In all of these clinics, patient satisfaction was high, which suggests that patients may not be very sensitive to the quality of data collection by the clinicians and their relationship with them is more important. In the conventional clinic, the patients spent less time in clinic overall, although on average the time difference was small. In the computerised clinic there were small reductions in the time spent examining the patient, and more time writing or typing. Doctors spent more time instructing the patient and there was less time with the patient giving information (Figure 12.3). Superficially the latter two observations could raise concern but this was largely a result of the fact that the doctor had already acquired much of the essential information and, therefore, the consultation was given 'a jump start'. With serial visits a clear indication of trends in morbidity could be discerned – one carrot (if not an irresistible one). Video analysis of the consultations showed no important differences in non-verbal communication.

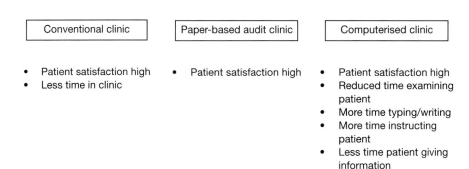

Figure 12.3 Impact of computerisation of an asthma clinic (King et al. 1993).

Development of a lung cancer audit tool (Kaltenthaler 2001)

This paper describes an ambitious process for development of a lung cancer audit tool that was designed to be comprehensive, covering all of the components of a clinical service. The project started from scratch: relevant standards were identified by performing a literature review and by consulting expert professionals for sources of appropriate documentation. This was then backed up by interviews with relevant healthcare professionals, followed by identification of information given by the literature review and interviews (Figure 12.4). The information identified included that being currently collected, that which should be collected, and also details of how, when, where and by whom the data should be collected. It was found, not surprisingly, that data would be collected in the settings of primary, secondary and tertiary care, as well as palliative care and purely in informatics. Audit forms were then designed for these separate areas. These were given trials, modified and implemented (Figure 12.4).

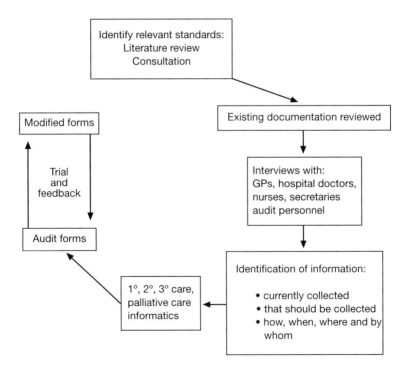

Figure 12.4 Development of a lung cancer audit tool.

In this model the 'good idea' demonstrated by the previous two examples was not employed, i.e. patients were not data collectors. Figure 12.5 shows, in the left-hand column, the patient pathway and, in the right, the people responsible for completing the audit form. It is apparent that the clinician and medical secretary are responsible for most of the data collection. This reflects what happens in the usual clinical process and reflects the method by which the audit tool was developed. However, although medical secretaries are good at following protocols and adjusting their work patterns, this does not tend to be the case for clinicians. This is perhaps reflected in the results of the study (Taenzer et al. 2000):

- 54 patients referred, 53 allocated forms
- initial page completed by medical secretary (100%)
- preclinical forms completed in 68%
- record of multidisciplinary meeting (MDT) decision in 42%
- all chemo- and radiotherapy forms completed retrospectively
- no surgical forms completed
- limited to a 3-month trial period.

Unfortunately, in the published version, the follow-up period was limited to a 3-month trial period only but nevertheless showed that, although the initial page was completed by the medical secretary in all allocated forms, the rest of the forms were not. Some forms were completed retrospectively, which requires extra time and personnel and where possible should be avoided.

This study illustrates an exemplary process of developing an audit tool but unfortunately does not address the difficult issues relating to methodology if data collection is to be 'built in'. Where possible the amount of clinician time involved in data entry should be reduced, because clinicians are very poor at collecting data. However, even if one has a whole army of audit personnel following the clinician around, those essential clinical data will still be incomplete. If the data are made essential to clinical management and the opportunity for collecting them is presented, then this problem will be minimised.

The next example illustrates integration of data collection with a clinical service and, although it is not able to provide the same comprehensive information, it does provide real-time data verification and built in data collection.

Integration and verification: focus on the multidisciplinary meeting

This example is applicable to the clinical services of many hospitals dealing with all types of tumour because Calman–Hine cancer service models focus on the multidisciplinary approach to management of cancer. This has inevitably led to the development of MDT meetings where management options are discussed before presenting these options to the patient. Nottingham City Hospital is a large teaching

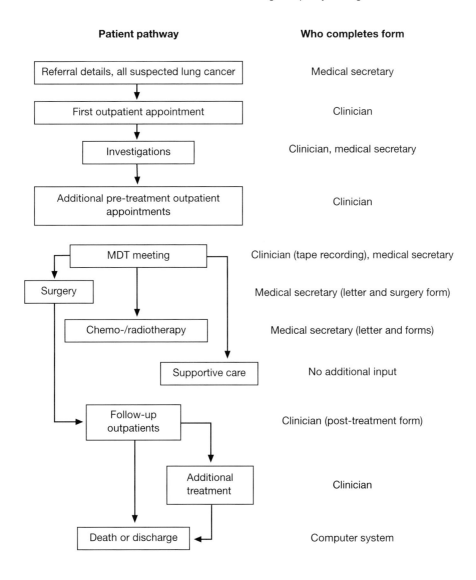

Patient pathway | **Who completes form**

Referral details, all suspected lung cancer — Medical secretary

First outpatient appointment — Clinician

Investigations — Clinician, medical secretary

Additional pre-treatment outpatient appointments — Clinician

MDT meeting — Clinician (tape recording), medical secretary

Surgery — Medical secretary (letter and surgery form)

Chemo-/radiotherapy — Medical secretary (letter and forms)

Supportive care — No additional input

Follow-up outpatients — Clinician (post-treatment form)

Additional treatment — Clinician

Death or discharge — Computer system

Figure 12.5 Lung cancer tool: 12 separate forms.

hospital and sees around 200 new lung cancer patients each year. Most of the patients are referred to the respiratory medicine service where the relevant investigations are organised to provide sufficient information for diagnosis and management. The patients are then presented at a multiprofessional meeting, and straight after this a multidisciplinary clinic is held where the patient's results are explained and the management options set before them (Figure 12.6). The patient is then referred to the appropriate service for therapy (usually available on the same day). Behind this clinical management process is one essential extra duty (Figure 12.7). Before presenting the patient at the multidisciplinary summary and at the same time as the patient is referred to the specialist multidisciplinary lung cancer clinic, a paper form is completed by a clinician. The paper form corresponds to a series of database fields which are entered by a lung oncology coordinator on to a simple database. From this database, a hard copy is generated and attached to the case notes with the original beneath it. The clinician, often the same one who has completed the form, then presents the clinical scenario at the MDT meeting with reference to the hard copy. This is the first opportunity for real-time data verification, confirming both that the information held on the database is correct and that the detail of information is sufficient. The form is then modified during the meeting, including such essential items as clinical stage and a further hard copy generated and attached to the case notes. The form may then be further modified after consultation with the patient to include items such as words used in explaining options to the patient. The form is then faxed directly to the general practitioner.

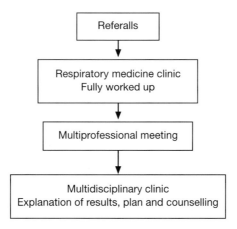

Figure 12.6 Integration and verification: focus on multidisciplinary team (MDT) meeting.

Perhaps one of the most rewarding aspects of this system has been the response of the GPs to receiving this level of information quickly and efficiently. Some patients, even when they have seen clinicians in the lung cancer clinic, still go back to their GP for explanations and GPs find such timely information invaluable in these circumstances.

From an information technology point of view, this system illustrates how 'built in' data collection can be and how real-time data verification *by clinicians* can be

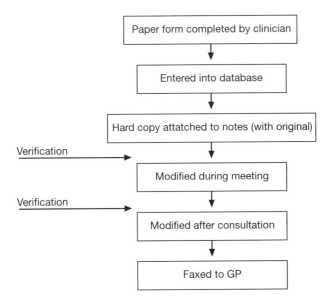

Figure 12.7 Integration and verification: focus on multidisciplinary team (MDT) meeting.

achieved. The crucial feature is that data collection has become part of clinical management with minimal disruption to the process. Essential data are now discussed at the meeting (e.g. lung function) whereas previously it would be relatively easy to miss these data for some patients.

Relevant outcomes – towards formal accreditation of lung cancer services

Careful definition of datasets, attention to methodology and clinical sponsorship should lead to relevant and accurate information. Potentially, there could be an explosion of information and it is important therefore that outcomes are clearly defined so that they may be compared across services. Some datasets include suggested outcome criteria (Thompson et al. 1999). Performance can be measured against predefined standards and accreditation can move to a new level. Thus far the cancer accreditation process has been about ensuring that the necessary infrastructure is in place to provide equitable cancer services, but what is really required is a measure of the comparative performance of services corrected for all of the important confounding variables. It is important that conclusions are not drawn from small statistically irrelevant samples, including small audits that do not stand up to statistical tests. Outcomes should ideally reflect the pyramid of data collection (see Figure 12.1) and, if there are no important differences using relatively few data, then further interrogation should occur only if there are good reasons to suspect that important differences are being concealed by combining subgroups. This will minimise the tendency for the management of healthcare information to become an end in itself (Wyatt and Keen 2001).

Conclusions

At last there are strong driving forces for healthcare data collection and the real possibility that healthcare information will catch up on its traditional 5-year lag behind industry (Wallace 1994). However, it is essential that this drive does not lead to the collection of data of insufficient quality. The challenge is to collect relevant, accurate and complete data that are readily accessible and provide appropriate outcomes to measure quality of care. The mechanism for data collection has already started in the development of important minimum datasets that include lung cancer. There is also recognition that resources must be channelled into data collection, including the development of an audit infrastructure, and recognition that data collectors are an essential part of a clinical management team. The development of clinical data collection in lung cancer, as with many areas of healthcare technology, is piecemeal and there are examples of good practice, although they are not comprehensive. The methodology for clinical data collection must be robust and sustainable, and must exhibit the essential features of real-time verification and full integration with the clinical service. In these developing phases, the whole process must be supported with determined and sustained clinical sponsorship.

References

Department of Health (1998) *Information for Health*. London: Department of Health.

Department of Health (2001) *Building the Information Core: Implementing the NHS plan*. London: Department of Health.

Fergusson RJ, Gregor A, Dodds R, Kerr G (1996) Management of lung cancer in South East Scotland. *Thorax* **51**: 569–574.

Gilligan D (1998) Recent developments in the diagnosis and treatment of lung cancer. *International Journal of Clinical Practice* **52**: 330–333.

Kaltenthaler E, McDonnell A, Peters J (2001) Monitoring the care of lung cancer patients: linking audit and care pathways. *Journal of Evaluation in Clinical Practice* **7**: 13–20.

King R, Baldwin DR, Pantin CFA (1993) The introduction of a written questionnaire based auditing system does not prolong the consultation times at an asthma clinic. *European Respiratory Journal* **17**: 145s.

NHS Executive (1998) *Guidance on Commissioning Cancer Services. Improving outcomes in lung cancer: The Manual*. Leeds: NHS Executive.

Royal College of Radiologists' Clinical Oncology Information Network (1999) Guidelines on the non-surgical management of lung cancer. *Clinical Oncology* **11**: S1–S53.

Scottish Intercollegiate Guidelines Network (1998) Management of lung cancer (http://pc47.ccc.hw.ac.uk/sing/home.htm).

Taenzer P, Bultz BD, Carlson LE et al. (2000) Impact of computerised quality of life screening on physician behaviour and patient satisfaction in lung cancer outpatients. *Psychooncology* **9**: 203–213.

Thompson S, Peake M, Macbeth F, Pearson M (eds) (1999) *Lung Cancer. A core dataset for the measurement of process and outcome in lung cancer management.* London: Royal College of Physicians.

Wallace S (1994) *The Computerised Patient Record.* Byte CMP: United Business Media.

Wyatt JC, Keen J (2001) New NHS Information Technology Strategy. Technology will change practice. *British Medical Journal* **322**: 1378–1379.

Index